Praise for *The Holistic Gui*

"Wow! What a good gut-health read. Dr. Mark, one of America's most trusted doctors, takes you on an easy-reading journey through your gut. As an experienced and science-based author, Dr. Stengler uses memorable phrases and engaging infographics to 'show and tell' you how to enjoy his life's teaching: better gut health, better total-body health. My wish for you wise readers: learn it, do it, and feel it. I personally have followed his good-gut-health plan and am enjoying vibrant head-brain and gut-brain health."

— **William Sears, M.D.**, best-selling author of multiple books, including *The Healthy Brain Book*

"A brilliant exposé on the true and devastating impact of the leaky gut on the entire body. Dr. Stengler has done it again: he has deciphered and demystified the true health impact of a 'leaky gut.' The gut is so much more than the epicenter of digestion. It is the first line of defense and protection from the outside world. Each day we fuel our bodies with food and drink, and we depend on the innate wisdom and integrity of our GI tract and the microbiome to moderate and mitigate what enters our bloodstream and inner workings. Expanding on the concept of leaky gut–leaky brain, Dr. Mark gives you a play-by-play on how a leaky gut impacts each cell of your body. This book is a must-have to know the real truth about leaky gut and overall gut health."

— **Chris Meletis, N.D.**, author of *The Disciples' Diet*

"Dr. Stengler shares the research and physiology behind leaky gut syndrome with expertise. This book is written in such a way that patients, physicians, and other healthcare providers alike can learn about leaky gut syndrome and dysbiosis."

— **Linette Williamson, M.D., ABAARM**

THE

HOLISTIC

GUIDE

TO GUT

HEALTH

ALSO BY DR. MARK STENGLER

*Healing the Prostate: The Best Holistic Methods
to Treat the Prostate and Other Common Male-Related Conditions**

Outside the Box Cancer Therapies
(with Dr. Paul Anderson)*

Prescription for Drug Alternatives
(with James Balch, M.D., and Robin Young Balch, N.D.)

The Natural Physician's Healing Therapies

Prescription for Natural Cures
(with James Balch, M.D., and Robin Young Balch, N.D.)

*Available from Hay House

Please visit:

Hay House USA: www.hayhouse.com®
Hay House Australia: www.hayhouse.com.au
Hay House UK: www.hayhouse.co.uk
Hay House India: www.hayhouse.co.in

THE

HOLISTIC GUIDE TO GUT HEALTH

Discover the Truth about Leaky Gut,
Balancing Your Microbiome,
and Restoring Whole-Body Health

Dr. Mark Stengler

HAY HOUSE, INC.
Carlsbad, California • New York City
London • Sydney • New Delhi

Published in the United States by: Hay House, Inc.: www.hayhouse.com®
Published in Australia by: Hay House Australia Pty. Ltd.: www.hayhouse.com.au
Published in the United Kingdom by: Hay House UK, Ltd.: www.hayhouse.co.uk
Published in India by: Hay House Publishers India: www.hayhouse.co.in

*Cover design: the*BookDesigners • *Interior design:* Karim J. Garcia
Indexer: Shapiro Indexing Services • *Interior illustrations:* Images used under
license from Shutterstock.com

Cataloging-in-Publication Data is on file with the Library of Congress

Tradepaper ISBN: 978-1-4019-7510-4
E-book ISBN: 978-1-4019-7511-1
Audiobook ISBN: 978-1-4019-7512-8

10 9 8 7 6 5 4 3 2 1
1st edition, April 2024

Printed in the United States of America

This product uses papers sourced from responsibly managed forests. For more information, see www.hayhouse.com.

*To all those looking to
treat digestive ailments and
the root cause of disease.*

CONTENTS

FOREWORD

As an integrative gastroenterologist who is also board certified in gastroenterology and internal medicine, I can attest that gut health is essential for overall health and wellness. In my research and writings, I have outlined the direct connection between whole body health and the health of the gut microbiome and digestive system. For this reason, I was very pleased to read Dr. Stengler's scientific and holistic approach to the gut-body connection in this book, *The Holistic Guide to Gut Health*. I wholeheartedly agree with Dr. Stengler that leaky gut syndrome and microbiome imbalance are commonly at the root of digestive and systemic health problems. This book is an important guide for anyone who wants to learn and understand more about this.

My mission is to help patients prevent and heal digestive ailments. This requires modern diagnostic tests, examining the patient, and the correct use of pharmaceutical and surgical therapies, which I know Dr. Stengler also endorses. However, early in my medical career, I noticed something was missing from my conventional medical training. This led me to learn about integrative medicine, which highlights nutritional and other natural therapies that promote body healing, so I could add to the toolbox of options I have as a doctor. I found that this approach was the missing link for safe and effective results for my patients. Moreover, I was fortunate to undergo extensive training in integrative medicine and become a diplomate of the American Board of Integrative Medicine.

I am a big proponent of the use of diet and targeted nutritional supplements for digestive healing. I use these natural therapies with patients as sole treatments as well as in combination with conventional therapies. I have witnessed the dramatic effectiveness of optimizing nutrition in my own health and that of thousands of my patients.

In *The Holistic Guide to Gut Health*, Dr. Stengler incorporates good science and practical, integrative therapies for the best all-around care for his readers and patients. For anyone interested in understanding how to optimize gut health, this book is an important resource.

— Marvin Singh, M.D.,
founder of Precisione Clinic,
author of *Rescue Your Health: How New Advances in Science Can Help You Feel Better, Boost Performance, and Live Longer*,
and co-author of *Integrative Gastroenterology: Second Edition*
www.precisioneclinic.com and www.rescueyourhealth.com

INTRODUCTION

The digestive tract contains intricately designed organs involved in the digestion and absorption of food required for life-giving energy and body repair. It also serves as the primary source of the trillions of microbes known as the *gut microbiome,* which play a critical role in digestion and immunity. In many ways, the digestive tract, especially the small intestine, is the primary region of the body that acts as a gateway for preventing or causing disease.

Leaky gut syndrome and dysbiosis are widespread conditions poorly addressed by the medical community. This book provides overwhelming scientific evidence in an easy-to-understand manner for how these digestive imbalances are enormous contributors to common and uncommon diseases, poor vitality, and aging. First, you will discover how to identify leaky gut syndrome and dysbiosis. Then, using my scientific and clinically proven holistic methods, you will learn how to use diet, supplements, and lifestyle choices to support digestion and absorption and heal a leaky gut and dysbiosis. This will benefit those with digestive conditions as well as those with conditions affecting other systems, since the digestive tract is interconnected with virtually all systems of the body.

WHY I WROTE THIS BOOK

While medical technology continues to improve in the United States, the number of people with chronic disease conditions is simultaneously increasing, with nearly 60 percent of all adults managing some form of chronic illness.[1] In addition, more than 35 million doctor visits yearly are due to digestive problems. These two health trends have a strong connection: poor gut health is directly or indirectly linked to most chronic health problems. Unfortunately, the health profession is largely ignorant of the gut-body connection. Instead, practitioners who go beyond the mainstream medical system have led the charge in addressing gut problems and whole-body health. Thanks to integrative, natu-ropathic, and functional doctors, as well as nutrition-oriented practitioners, many people with a wide variety of chronic health problems have found relief by addressing the root issues of leaky gut and dysbiosis.

The widespread problems of leaky gut and dysbiosis are best addressed with holistic healing methods, not drugs and surgery. This fact makes many doctors incapable of helping with these conditions, even if they know how to diagnose them. I wrote this book to help the public and healthcare professionals understand the science behind leaky gut and dysbiosis and the best treatments for prevention and recovery.

The Holistic Guide to Gut Health is designed to be a compre-hensive yet user-friendly guidebook that illuminates the most effective therapies for leaky gut syndrome, dysbiosis, common digestive ailments, and whole-body health related to the digestive tract. It's important to communicate with your doctor regarding any protocols you wish to put into practice, especially for serious illnesses like cancer. Proper monitoring is essential for the best health outcomes. For the most up-to-date health news, recom-mendations, and further resources to help you explore the topics in this book, please visit my website: www.markstengler.com.

All my best,
Mark Stengler, N.M.D., M.S.

PART I

IT'S ALL
ABOUT
THE GUT

Chapter 1

GUT HEALTH IS
WHOLE-BODY HEALTH

Susan, a 35-year-old Internet marketer, suffered from irritable bowel syndrome (IBS) and fatigue for more than 10 years. It began in college, when her stress level was high and her diet consisted of mainly fast food. She had thought her low energy level was due to all the stress, but her chiropractor suggested that leaky gut syndrome might be at the root of many of her health issues. When Susan consulted with her family medical doctor about the possibility of having leaky gut syndrome, her doctor rolled her eyes and said this was a condition that only "very sick" people have. After reading some of my articles on the topic, Susan scheduled a visit with me. I told her that leaky gut was indeed a true medical condition and that she had many of the common symptoms. A blood test confirmed the diagnosis, and I placed her on my leaky gut healing protocol. Susan experienced noticeable improvement in her digestive symptoms within just 10 days. Then, at the three-week mark, her energy began improving and continued to improve, along with her digestive symptoms. After eight weeks she reported that she had the digestion and energy of her teen years. She could not believe the improvement.

As you can see from Susan's story, if you want to have whole-body health, then you must have a healthy gut. The health of your gut affects all organs and cells of your body, including your brain, skin, heart, liver, muscles, joints, eyes, immune system, and more. As a result, your energy, mood, memory, weight and metabolism, muscle and joint health, resistance to autoimmunity or infection, and hormone balance are all related to your gut health. The connection between gut health and the rest of the body makes sense when you consider all the activities occurring in the digestive system. The simple fact is that all your cells need nutrients to survive and function, and most of that nutrition comes from what you consume and then absorb through your gut. The health of your gut can either be your gateway to excellent health and vitality . . . or a direct route to poor health and disease.

Your gut is also the epicenter of much of your immune system. If you want to have more resiliency to infection or be less prone to autoimmunity—and even cancer—then you must have a healthy digestive system. Another important aspect of gut health is the microbiome. The balance between the various microbes in your gut has a tremendous influence on whole-body health, and I will explain what this means and how you can best support your microbiome.

In this book, you will learn the truth about the gut-body connection and what you can do to resolve this fundamental root cause of so many health problems. There is one essential fact you will come to understand: The health of your gut directly affects whether you are healthy or sick!

COMMON MYTHS

Before we go any further, let me dispel some common myths regarding the relationship between digestive health and whole-body health. You may have read these myths in books, learned them in your high school or college biology classes, or read them online.

Myth #1: There is no medical ailment known as a leaky gut.

Anyone who claims there is no such thing as a leaky gut is out of touch with the latest scientific research. As you will read later in this chapter, there is a tremendous amount of evidence that leaky gut is not only real but also quite common. Doctors who do not recognize leaky gut as a medical condition are missing the root cause of many of their patient's health problems.

Myth #2: Natural therapies do not help leaky gut.

Nothing could be further from the truth. There are natural therapies shown to heal leaky gut and help in the healing of many digestive ailments, and they are by far the best way to treat and prevent leaky gut. The correct healing foods and supplements as well as good lifestyle habits, such as exercise, stress reduction, and proper sleep, provide the basis for gut healing. There is also strong scientific research on dietary and supplemental approaches to healing leaky gut. These natural approaches have the benefit of treating the root causes of leaky gut and digestive disorders. The problem our medical system has when it comes to treating digestive ailments with holistic and nutritional approaches is that most doctors have no training in this field. Fortunately, there are a growing number of naturopathic medical doctors, integrative doctors, functional medical practitioners, and holistic healthcare providers in North America and globally who are trained in the proper diagnosis and treatment of leaky gut and common digestive ailments.

Myth #3: Toxins from the digestive tract do not get absorbed into the bloodstream.

Many conventional doctors claim that toxins are not readily absorbed from the small intestine or large intestine except in rare cases of severe gut illness, but the scientific literature reveals that toxins are in fact absorbed from the small intestine into the bloodstream. In addition, bacterial toxins that should be eliminated by the colon can be reabsorbed from the colon into the bloodstream.

Naturopathic doctors and holistic practitioners have historically referred to this as toxemia.

Myth #4: Drugs and surgery are the only ways to treat digestive issues.

While there are pharmaceutical and surgical procedures for certain digestive problems, there are many effective natural approaches as well that should almost always be implemented, especially for chronic digestive issues. There are times when drugs and surgery are required along with natural approaches. Specialists in digestive diseases are known as gastroenterologists. However, few gastroenterologists have much training in nutritional and integrative approaches to digestive healing. This book will discuss the dietary and natural approaches to treating common digestive problems.

Myth #5: Improving gut microbiome balance is only for people with digestive problems.

The gut microbiome is connected to all the systems of the body. Therefore gut problems such as dysbiosis have the potential to cause imbalances in other organ systems. Moreover, a modern approach to preventing and treating health disorders begins with improving the health of the gut microbiome. Since we are now in an era of precision medicine, a well-rounded doctor will assess and treat dysbiosis (and leaky gut) for patients with most conditions.

ANCIENT HEALING SYSTEMS AND DIGESTIVE HEALING

Ancient healers have long acknowledged that the health of the digestive tract dramatically affects the health of the whole body. Many healing systems, including Traditional Chinese Medicine (TCM), Ayurveda, South American herbalism (such as those practices found in the Amazon region), European and North American

Naturopathic medicine, and most natural healing systems throughout the world, recognize the vital link between digestive health and whole-body health. The gut-body connection is part of the larger holistic premise that health and healing are generally prioritized from the inside to the outside of the body. And, of course, the core of the inside of your body is the digestive tract!

TCM has long appreciated the relationship between the digestive organs and their effect on other body organs. Diet, massage, moxibustion, and acupuncture are used to balance the digestive organs and thus establish harmony with other organ systems of the body. Ayurvedic medicine, which is common in India and increasingly popular in the United States, takes a similar balancing approach to digestive organs to improve whole-body health. These ancient systems take into account different types of imbalances within the organ system and have detailed therapies to address these imbalances, such as using certain foods and herbs.

European holistic medicine has a rich history of understanding the importance of digestive function and its connection to whole-body health. For example, they value using digestive herbal tonics, particularly bitter herbs, as a treatment for improving digestive function and therefore treating chronic diseases. Hydrotherapy—the use of hot and cold water to stimulate nerve and blood flow to the digestive organs—is another ancient treatment. These therapies are still in use today in countries such as Germany, Switzerland, England, and Russia, as well as in other regions of Europe.

Tens of thousands of North American holistic and integrative doctors have acknowledged that their clinical experience correlates with the published scientific research on leaky gut syndrome. The science of identifying and treating leaky gut is a normal part of the curriculum for naturopathic medical doctors, integrative doctors, TCM practitioners and acupuncturists, chiropractors, holistic nutritionists, and functional medicine practitioners. Unfortunately, you would be hard-pressed to find the academic curriculum and continuing education training for typical healthcare providers to include training on leaky gut and holistic approaches to common digestive ailments.

MODERN MEDICINE NEEDS TO MODERNIZE

Until recently, much of conventional medicine attempted to discredit the ancient notion of gut health imbalance and its association with digestive and non-digestive illness. Now medical researchers and gastroenterologists at the forefront of gut permeability research have done a complete turnaround and acknowledge the medical reality of "leaky gut." Simply put, leaky gut (increased intestinal permeability) occurs when the small intestine lining is damaged by a variety of factors (diet, stress, medications, toxins, infections, and others). As a result, there is increased permeability to substances that should not penetrate the intestinal barrier, and two things occur: First, there is an immune and inflammatory reaction in the intestinal cells, which causes localized damage; second, molecules that should not be absorbed through the gut wall make their way into the bloodstream. The immune system reacts with an inflammatory response, which can then affect other areas of the body in an adverse fashion. According to the *Journal of the Endocrine Society*, "Intestinal barrier function is critical for normal homeostasis of the gut, and the breakdown or dysfunction of this barrier is associated with local as well as systemic consequences largely related to direct contact of bacteria/bacterial products with the epithelial cells, and translocation of these to the systemic circulation."[1]

As modern scientific research has proven, ancient healers and today's integrative doctors were correct about leaky gut. For example, Harvard Health Publishing published an article recognizing the legitimacy of leaky gut and noted that most doctors would not recognize the term.[2] In a separate article the same publisher stated this about leaky gut:

> The lining of the intestine is made of millions and millions of cells. These cells join together to create a tight barrier that acts like a security system and decides what gets absorbed into the bloodstream and what stays out. However, when the gut becomes unhealthy, the lining can weaken, so "holes" develop in the barrier. The result is that toxins and bacteria can leak into

the bloodstream. This can trigger inflammation in the gut and throughout the body and cause a chain reaction of problems, such as bloating, gas, cramps, food sensitivities, fatigue, headaches, and joint pain, to name a few.[3]

Another article in the mainstream medical journal *Frontiers in Immunology* revealed, "Disruption of the epithelial barrier increases intestinal permeability, resulting in leaky gut syndrome (LGS)."[4] The epithelial layer refers to the cells that line the small intestine.

Many experts agree that leaky gut occurs in conditions such as inflammatory bowel disease (e.g., Crohn's disease), irritable bowel syndrome (IBS), and celiac disease. However, research also indicates that leaky gut increases in various other diseases, such as diabetes, chronic kidney disease, cancer, and cardiovascular diseases. Moreover, recent research has shown that a leaky gut is a common occurrence with aging. Finally, integrative doctors like myself have found that leaky gut can occur in a less severe disease state.

Dysbiosis goes hand in hand with a leaky gut. Dysbiosis refers to an imbalance of the gut microbiota with reduced beneficial microbes and increased pathogenic microbes. It results from the processed American diet, medications such as antibiotics and acid reflux drugs, and high stress levels. Modern medicine acknowledges dysbiosis but does little to address this significant health problem associated with a leaky gut.

Unfortunately, many doctors are unaware of the all-too-common problems of leaky gut and dysbiosis. As a result, the root cause of your health problems may not be addressed. You may receive a prescription to help with your uncomfortable symptoms, but real healing at a deeper level will not occur. The good news is that this book will give you far more understanding than the average medical doctor on this critically important health subject.

Dr. Alessio Fasano is a pediatric gastroenterologist who has published a summary of chronic inflammatory diseases related to leaky gut.[5] His list includes:

- aging
- ankylosing spondylitis
- attention deficit hyperactivity disorder (ADHD)
- autism
- celiac disease and non-celiac gluten sensitivity
- chronic fatigue syndrome/myalgic encephalomyelitis
- colitis/inflammatory bowel diseases
- environmental enteric dysfunction
- gestational diabetes
- glioma
- insulin resistance
- irritable bowel syndrome (IBS)
- HIV
- hyperlipidemia
- major depressive disorders
- multiple sclerosis
- necrotizing enterocolitis
- nonalcoholic fatty liver disease
- obesity
- schizophrenia
- sepsis
- type 1 diabetes
- type 2 diabetes

But there is more! *Nature Reviews Immunology* reported evidence for the following additional conditions connected to leaky gut:[6]

- allergic rhinitis (hay fever)
- Alzheimer's disease
- asthma

- atopic dermatitis (eczema)
- autoimmune hepatitis
- chronic depression
- chronic rhinosinusitis (nasal and sinus inflammation)
- eosinophilic esophagitis
- liver cirrhosis
- occupational asthma and chronic bronchitis[6]
- Parkinson's disease
- rheumatoid arthritis
- stress-related psychiatric disorders
- systemic lupus erythematosus

You can see that mainstream medical literature has recognized all these diseases associated with leaky gut. So why have none of your medical professionals told you about this?

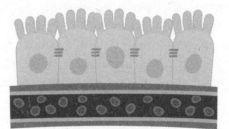

Normal tight junction

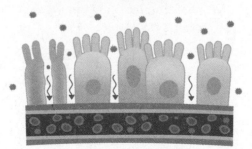

Leaky and inflamed

Image 1.1: Leaky Gut

YOUR INNER WORKINGS

The digestive system is an engineering masterpiece that harnesses life-giving nutrients and water from your diet. Let's take a closer look at this amazing system and its subsystems.

When you eat, the food is mechanically broken down by chewing (assuming you take the time to chew your food) and then chemically broken down with enzymes in saliva (for carbohydrates and fat). The food then moves into the stomach, where protein is broken down by the action of the enzyme pepsin (which is activated by hydrochloric acid). The stomach also produces lipase, which is an enzyme that breaks down fat.

Next your food travels to the small intestine, the digestive tube found between the stomach and the large intestine (colon), where most of the absorption of nutrients occurs. Food (carbohydrates, fats, and proteins) is chemically broken down for digestion and absorption in the small intestine by digestive enzymes secreted by the pancreas. Bile made in the liver and stored in the gallbladder mixes with food in the small intestine for fat digestion. The small intestine also contains specialized cells known as *brush border enzymes* that synthesize enzymes that help digest food. And last, the small intestine cells known as enteroendocrine cells produce several hormones that act as chemical messengers to stimulate the activation of digestive secretions in the stomach, pancreas, and gallbladder.

The last area of digestion is the colon, where some water is reabsorbed, minerals such as sodium and chloride can be absorbed, and the remaining fecal material is excreted out of the body through the rectum.

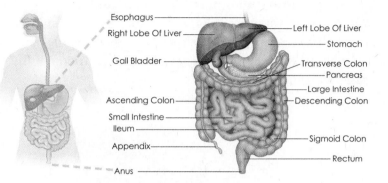

Image 1.2: The Digestive System

The Sensational Small Intestine

The small intestine is approximately 28 feet of tubing between the stomach and large intestine. The mucosal lining is composed of unique folds and projections known as villi. The combination of these folds increases the absorptive area by up to 120 times.[7] It is amazing to recognize that the small intestine's surface area is as large as 400m², which is equal to about two tennis courts![8] The gastrointestinal tract receives 60 tons of food over a lifetime.[9] It plays a critical role in the exchange between the body, microbiome (bacteria in the gut), and body exposure to foreign substances through intestinal absorption.

But the small intestine is much more than a hollow tube. It is composed of several layers and specialized structures and chemicals that work in synergy to protect against infection and damage, while also providing a route for nutrients to be absorbed into the body.

There are three main regions of the small intestine: the duodenum, the jejunum, and the ileum. The duodenum is the shortest section of the small intestine and where chemical digestion with digestive juices and enzymes takes place. It begins at the lower end of the stomach and connects to the jejunum. The jejunum continues to mix the food. It contains projections known as villi, which are involved in the absorption of glucose, amino acids, calcium, iron, folate, fats and fat soluble vitamins, sodium, and water. It empties into the last portion of the small intestine, the ileum. The ileum also has villi, and is involved in the absorption of B12, bile acid, water, and sodium.[10]

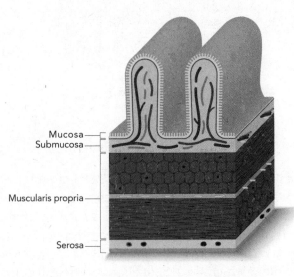

Image 1.3: The Layers of the Small Intestine

The small intestine also has four main layers. Describing them in order from the outermost to the innermost layer:[11]

- The **serosa** layer contains the outermost lining of the small intestine and the all-important epithelium.

- The **muscularis propria** are two layers of smooth muscle and the nerves between the two layers.

- The **submucosa** is a layer of connective tissue that contains blood vessels, nerves, and lymphatics.

- The **mucosa** is the innermost layer of the small intestine that contains enterocytes with villi that are involved with absorption, goblet cells, and enteroendocrine cells.

Lastly and very importantly for our discussion on leaky gut, the intestinal barrier has four layers:[12]

Layer 1

The first and top layer includes the luminal *intestinal alkaline phosphatase* (IAP). IAP is a protein or enzyme located in the inside space of the intestines as well as directly below in the second layer. The function of IAP is to break down the toxin *lipopolysaccharide* (LPS) from bacteria, which is known to cause gut inflammation and permeability. It also protects the small intestinal lining by regulating the proteins involved in controlling permeablity, the microbes in the small intestine, and the antimicrobial proteins that keep harmful bacteria from flourishing. IAP also induces the process of autophagy (death of old cells so new ones can form) and possibly plays a role in the synthesis of mucus in layer 2.[13]

Layer 2

The second layer is the *intestinal mucosal layer.* This layer acts as the first physical barrier to bacteria that can be dangerous to the digestive tract. There are two mucus layers: the inner layer prevents harmful bacteria (and other microbes) from penetrating the lining of the epithelial cells; the outer layer stores healthy bacteria that prevent disease-causing bacteria and microbes from entering into the mucus layer. These two mucus layers contain water, electrolytes, antibodies, and other substances. Mucus is secreted by specialized cells known as *goblet cells,* which are located in the epithelial cells.

Layer 3

The third layer is a continuous single layer of cells known as *intestinal epithelial cells* (IECs). This layer functions as a selective physical barrier for the small intestine by regulating what contents pass through into the bloodstream below. It prevents harmful substances such as toxins, microorganisms, and foreign proteins from entering, while allowing life-giving nutrients, electrolytes, and water to be absorbed into the bloodstream to be carried to cells of the body. The potential for substances to be absorbed across the intestinal lining depend on their size, hydrophobicity (i.e., repelled by water or not able to mix with water), and other physical and chemical properties.[14]

The natural barrier of the small intestine is designed to prevent bacteria, fungi, and other microbes, as well as undigested food particles or foreign particles, from entering the bloodstream. This physical barrier is also known as the *intestinal epithelial barrier function* (IEBF). When the IEBF becomes compromised, it can lead to a breakdown in the gut and the whole body. As *Marine Drugs* explains, "Compromised IEBF has been associated with several pathological conditions, both intestinal and systemic, such as inflammatory bowel diseases (IBDs), metabolic disorders, systemic inflammatory response syndrome (SIRS), etc."[15]

The contact between the IECs is sealed by what are known as *tight junctions*. There are at least seven types of IECs that have specialized functions. Epithelial cells also line the villi, allowing the absorption of nutrients into a network of capillaries and lymphatic vessels to be distributed throughout the body. The IECs are constantly being replaced with new cells and are renewed every three to five days due to stem cells located in the inward folds of the villi called *crypts*.

A regulated absorption system occurs between small intestine cells, known as the *paracellular pathway*. This pathway has spaces between IECs, which are regulated by more than 50 proteins making up the tight junctions. The tight junctions contain a number of protein structures that act as links adjoining epithelial cells. The tight junctions are dynamic in that they adapt to various circumstances (developmental, physiological, and pathological).[16] For example, when exposed to food poisoning, the proteins of the tight junctions change to allow the bacteria to pass through the gut instead of causing constant damage. Then the proteins adapt back to the normal pattern and allow the tighten the junction to return to a normal state. Items normally absorbed through the paracellular route include ions, water, and large hydrophilic (i.e., attracted to water and able to mix with water) compounds.[17]

The other absorptive pathway critical to life is the *transcellular pathway*. This pathway involves absorption within the small intestinal cells (enterocytes) instead of between cells (paracellular). The transcellular pathway is involved in the absorption of nutrients, including sugars, amino acids, and vitamins. This type of absorption requires transport carriers and energy. Leaky gut can occur in the increased permeability of both pathways.

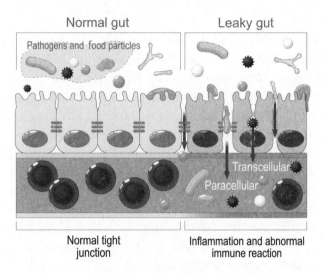

Image 1.4: Leaky Gut Permeability of Pathways

A family of proteins known as *zonulin* are synthesized by intestinal cells (as well as other organs) and function to regulate gut permeability. When intestinal cells are exposed to pathogenic microbes (bad bacteria or other microbes), zonulin is released to open up the paracellular tight junctions to rid the gut of the toxin. Zonulin is also released when people have a gluten allergy (celiac) or non-celiac gluten sensitivity. This action is reversible so gut permeability is not constant. However, chronic exposure to agents that damage the intestinal lining leads to gut inflammation, systemic inflammation, and increased disease risk. High levels of zonulin in the stool and blood are associated with leaky gut problems.

In diagrams of the small intestine you will often see the term *lamina propria*. This is a layer of connective tissue that separates epithelial cells from a layer of smooth muscle. This tissue contains blood vessels and lymphatics that absorb the products of digestion as well as supply blood flow to and from the epithelial layer. The lamina propria also contains a variety of immune cells that fight infectious intruders.

Layer 4

This layer is found in the small intestinal crypts lined with IECs that contain specialized cells known as *paneth cells*. The paneth cells secrete antimicrobial peptides that play a role in immunity. The most plentiful of these peptides is alpha-defensin, which has antibacterial activity. Thus, layer 4 is technically referring to the antimicrobial peptides that have an antibacterial action. Also in layer 4 are stem cells, which are located in the intestinal crypts. Stem cells regenerate intestinal cells rapidly.[18] The production and activity of stem cells is important because intestinal epithelial cells are renewed every three to four days.[19] The paneth cells also have a regulating effect on stem cells. In addition, the fourth layer contains IgA antibodies, which attach to microorganisms and toxins to prevent infection, inflammation, and damage.

Consequences of Increased Intestinal Permeability

A breakdown in the integrity of the small intestine barrier results in local and systemic consequences. When microbial compounds come into contact with the epithelial cells, there is an activation from the local immune system within the area. Pro-inflammatory chemicals are released that cause localized inflammation. This localized inflammation in the gut can lead to the development of several gastrointestinal diseases.[20] In addition, the progression of leaky gut results in bacterial products such as lipopolysaccharides (LPS) getting into the bloodstream. This leads to a cascade of events in which pro-inflammatory compounds and immune cells are released and affect various parts of the body. The industrialized Western diet has been shown to cause leaky gut, which results in LPS being released into the bloodstream and systemic circulation, causing what is known as endotoxemia.[21]

Once these foreign particles come into contact with the small intestine, and even more so upon entering the bloodstream, the immune system responds to attack the intruders. As a result of the immune response, increased inflammation can affect the gut and the rest of the body. Also, an imbalanced immune response can make one more susceptible to infection or autoimmune disease.

The Marvelous Microbiome

When most people hear the word *microbiome*, they think of the digestive tract. However, the microbiome refers to the microorganisms in the gut and other areas of the human body. The microbiome encompasses many body areas, including the skin, urinary tract, vaginal region, and more. The microbiome is more than just bacteria—it includes fungi, protozoa, and viruses. Amazingly, the microbiome has an estimated 100 trillion microbes, most of which live in the gut.

You will see the terms *microbiome* and *microbiota* in different articles. Technically, microbiome refers to a microbial community that occupies a particular region and the activity of microorganisms, while microbiota refers to various microorganisms. The three main functions of the microbiome are to create metabolites used for energy, protect against disease-causing microbes, and regulate immunity.[22]

The human gut contains at least 1,000 different species of bacteria, with the two major categories known as *bacteroidetes* and *firmicutes*. The various organisms interact with one another in the microbiome. The gut microbiota account for an average of 3.3 to 4.4 pounds of fecal matter and contains about 150 times the number of human genes.[23] The gut microbiota produce a metabolite known as butyrate,[24] which has anti-inflammatory effects and prevents allergic diseases. Additional metabolites of gut bacterial fermentation that benefit the body include short-chain fatty acids such as acetate and propionate. These fatty acids protect against autoimmune and inflammatory reactions.

There is a symbiotic and complex relationship between the gut microbiome and the rest of the body. The microbiome plays a key role in developing cardiometabolic disease, intestinal inflammation, cancer, cognition, and neuropsychological disorders. *Nutrients* reported that: "The gut microbiome plays an important role in human health and influences the development of chronic diseases ranging from metabolic disease to gastrointestinal disorders and colorectal cancer."[25] Also, in medicine the microbiota is a therapeutic target for many of society's diseases.

The microbiome is now considered an essential organ of the body—and the largest organ of the body. It has many functions, including immunity, which provides defense against disease-causing pathogens; production of nutrients, such as short-chain fatty acids and vitamins; energy production; maintaining the intestinal lining; and even influencing your brain function. Your doctor performs a physical exam and lab tests to check your body's organs, but when was the last time they checked your microbiome organ health status? According to *Mayo Clinical Proceedings*, "The human microbiome is emerging as a key target of personalized medicine by offering interesting solutions for a variety of environmental and metabolic diseases."[26]

The human microbiome originates during pregnancy, when flora is transferred from the placenta, amniotic fluid, and meconium (first poop of a newborn baby) to the baby in the womb or after birth.[27] Research shows that infants delivered vaginally have higher amounts of gut bacteria compared to cesarean section. The same researchers note that colonization of the microbiome is critical the first week of life. Poor microbiota development during this time is correlated with increased risk of future conditions, such as cardiovascular disease and eczema (atopic disease). In addition, breast milk plays an important role in the healthy formation of the gut microbiota, including the important Bifidobacterium. In contrast, infants fed formula during the first month of life have fewer total number of gut bacteria species. The sugars in breast milk act as a prebiotic for healthy gut microbiota. As the child grows, their diet plays a significant role in the development of the gut microbiota.

The gut microbiome has a direct influence on gut wall integrity. Researchers have shown that the microbiome positively affects the gut lining through the upregulation of genes that produce mucin (natural mucus layer in the gut), production of the gut antibody known as IgA, cytokine (inflammatory chemical) secretion, suppression of intestinal inflammation, and restoration of the tight juncture structure. Alternatively, gut dysbiosis negatively affects intestinal permeability.

The role of dysbiosis in the microbiome is more common in people who are obese as compared to those who are lean. There is emerging evidence that gut dysbiosis plays a role in developing metabolic disorders such as obesity, type 2 diabetes, and nonalcoholic fatty liver disease, and the use of probiotics has demonstrated a decrease in body weight and body mass index (BMI) for those over 18. Regarding probiotic supplementation in those who are obese or overweight, the results have shown minor or no changes in body weight and BMI.

Two of the major causes of detrimental changes in the microbiome are the industrialized Western diet and the use of antibiotics. Antibiotics can have negative effects on the microbiota, including reduced diversity, antibiotic resistance, and susceptibility to various diseases.[28]

Improved genetic testing has allowed researchers to better understand what makes up a healthy microbiome. As you might expect, there is variation among individuals related to geographic locations and the foods they consume. The medical understanding of optimal microbiomes is still in development. However, researchers have come to some basic conclusions thus far on the human microbiome.[29] One item of importance is diversity. There are different types of diversity that can be analyzed, but for our purposes, diversity will refer to the different types of microbes in the gut as well as the families of microbes. It is thought that diversity generally correlates with greater resistance to disease, since reduced diversity can lead to the overgrowth of commensal bacteria. Commensal bacteria are a normal part of the gut flora, and the commensal gut microbiota protect the epithelial lining of the small intestine from being damaged by pathogenic microbes.[30] If there is overgrowth of the commensal bacteria, they can become disease causing.

As mentioned earlier, there are two main categories of bacteria known as firmicutes and bacteroidetes. The balance between these two is associated with some diseases. The gut microbiota vary depending on the region of the digestive tract. For example, the small intestine is less hospitable to microbes due to high bile concentration and relatively rapid transit time (compared to the large intestine). The large intestine has a slower transit time and milder acidic pH, and so contains the largest microbial community. The dominant type of bacteria species in the gut is related to your diet.[31]

The exact parameters of what constitutes a healthy gut microbiome are still being researched. According to an article in *Gastroenterology*, "As studies have progressively included larger numbers of human volunteers, it has become clear that the microbiome variance among apparently healthy individuals is vast. No single microbiome configuration is required for health; rather, various different configurations of the microbiome can be consistent with health."[32] The same authors note that although genetics play a role in our microbiome, the more dominant factors include environmental and lifestyle factors, ethnicity, geopgraphic location, diet, and medications used. Our microbiome is constantly changing throughout time as we age. There tends to be a loss of microbiota diversity as we grow older, which increases the risk of inflammation and frailty. The authors also emphasize that the simplest intervention for affecting the microbiome to reduce disease risk is diet. Moreover, according to *eLife*, the microbiome changes during aging because people are eating a less diverse diet and using medications. The journal also reported that younger people gain disease-associated microbes as they age, while older people have the tendency to lose healthy gut microbes.[33]

Microbiome testing by stool utilizes genetic testing, and reference ranges are provided by the laboratory. Imbalances or disease-causing microbes can be identified by these tests. However, since there is no consensus on precise parameters of these microbes, the quality of the testing and interpretation and recommendations given by a knowledgeable practitioner are paramount.

THE GUT-BODY CONNECTION

Science now recognizes that the gut, especially the small intestine and its microbiome, has a direct or indirect relationship and influence on the rest of the body's organs. For example, you can see how the small intestine and its role of absorption acts as a gateway for what enters the bloodstream, both good and bad. A plethora of research demonstrates that the gut microbiome is multidimensional and has a communication network with the major organ systems of the body.

When I am helping patients to heal, especially from chronic disease, I make sure that gut health is a priority for other parts of the body to heal. Gut health should always be on the mind of both the health practitioner and the patient, when creating an environment of healing. Here is a secret of the most successful integrative and holistic doctors and practitioners: they almost always focus on improving gut health to help their patients heal. I was fortunate to learn this early in my career, and now almost three decades later, I still rely on this principle.

THE IMPORTANT ROLE OF THE GUT IN IMMUNE HEALTH

Many people are concerned more than ever about the proper functioning of their immune system. People do not want to contract viruses like COVID-19, the flu, or other viral infections. Infections such as COVID-19 not only cause an acute infection but also are notorious for creating long-term symptoms, known as "long COVID" or "long haulers."

Infections like COVID-19 affect the gut. A meta-analysis of 50 studies of people with long COVID found that 22 percent experienced loss of appetite, dyspepsia (indigestion), irritable bowel syndrome, loss of taste, and abdominal pain.[34] Part of the reason that the gut is affected by long COVID is that there are ACE-2 receptors in the GI tract, which COVID spike proteins attach to and activate, possibly causing small intestinal cell inflammation and damage. In addition, the microbiome of people with long COVID had unhealthy changes in the gut flora, causing dysbiosis.

Jay, a 55-year-old executive, had been suffering from post-COVID fatigue for several months when I first saw him. His low energy was making it difficult to complete his work every day. His family doctor told him to "give it time," but Jay was getting increasingly concerned about his lack of improvement. As I took his history, I noticed that he was also suffering from gas and bloating, and occasional loose stool. I asked Jay if he had these digestive symptoms before COVID, and he said no. I told Jay that research had shown that COVID could cause an imbalance of the microbiome, and that the bacteria in the gut influence how cells produce energy and help manage body inflammation. I had Jay consume foods that worked as prebiotics to feed his good bacteria, as well as try probiotic meal planning that gave him direct sources of the good bacteria (there are many prebiotic and probiotic recipes at the end of this book). In addition, I had Jay supplement with a well-studied probiotic, digestive enzymes with meals, and turmeric extract to improve liver and gallbladder function and reduce body inflammation. Jay noticed improvement within two weeks, and within six weeks, his energy level was almost back to normal.

There are many infections besides COVID-19 that can affect gut health, which in turn compromise immune function. Some examples include Lyme disease, parasitic diseases like giardia, hepatitis, HIV, bacterial infections such as *Helicobacter pylori*, fungal infections such as *Candida albicans*, and others. The problem becomes cyclical when the gut is affected by the infection and causes symptoms, and then the immune system becomes compromised, which affects the body systemically.

To protect yourself against these microbes, I highly recommend that you get your gut health in order. One of the best long-term ways to have your immune system fight off infections is to have great gut health. There are many nutrients that the immune system requires to function properly, and a healthy digestive system will absorb the nutrients from food and supplements to supercharge your immune system. In addition, you will find out in the next chapter how specialized immune tissue in the gut powers your immune cells. And lastly, a damaged small intestine lining leads to abnormal immune function in the gut lining. This not only compromises your immune function for fighting off infections but also prevents your immune system from working properly to respond to many autoimmune diseases.

Chapter 2

YOUR GUT—THE ROOT OF ALL (YOUR) HEALTH PROBLEMS?

As you read in Chapter 1, the gut is a critical connection between the outside world and the internal environment of your body. Generally speaking, if you optimize your gut health, you set the stage for whole-body health. Therefore, if you want to prevent or heal from disease, you should make sure your gut is healthy.

Sonja, a 34-year-old executive, came to my clinic wanting to improve her thyroid function. She had been diagnosed with autoimmune thyroiditis, also known as Hashimoto's thyroiditis, a year earlier. Her thyroid levels were mildly low, so her functional doctor had her on a small amount of bioidentical thyroid. Sonja did not like the idea of being on thyroid replacement, even in small amounts. In taking her health history, I noticed that she had many symptoms of leaky gut and dysbiosis. Her history of using NSAIDs for a shoulder injury from volleyball was a large risk factor for leaky gut. Since she had had recovered from surgery, she no longer required NSAIDs. Blood tests confirmed a severe degree of leaky gut, and I placed her on my program. Her thyroid autoanti-bodies were retested after three months and showed a reduction of 70 percent. In addition, her own thyroid hormone levels increased without a change in her medication. At the six-month mark, her thyroid autoantibodies were in the normal range, and her leaky gut blood tests were normal. At this point I stopped her thyroid medication. We repeated her thyroid labs two months later and everything was normal. Sonja now completes blood work once a year and everything remains normal. Keeping her gut healthy has helped Sonja heal.

In this chapter, we'll review some of the major systems of the body, and I'll offer additional insight on how they are influ-enced by your gut. We'll explore your immune system, hormones, metabolism, brain and nervous system, musculoskeletal system, cardiovascular health, and more.

IMMUNITY

The immune system is an engineering marvel that consists of a network of organs and specialized cells and chemicals. The goal is to protect the outside and inside of your body from becoming a victim of infectious microbes. There is a direct connection between the health of your gut and the functioning of your immune sys-tem. Your intestinal lining contains numerous immune compo-nents, so problems like leaky gut and dysbiosis lead to an ongoing immune response, which creates inflammation and imbalance with the immune system. Your immune system also requires sev-eral nutrients for proper functioning, and absorption problems with leaky gut set the stage for nutrient deficiencies.

There has been a lot of research in recent years examining the link between leaky gut, dysbiosis, and autoimmunity. Foreign particles (toxins, pathogens, undigested food particles) that enter the epithelial lining of the small intestine cause a chain of events that turns the immune system against its own tissue.[1] As a result, many autoimmune diseases can occur, including type 1 diabetes, multiple sclerosis, inflammatory bowel disease, systemic lupus erythematosus, and others.

Another concern is the increased susceptibility to cancer. There is a relationship between cancer and inflammation, and gut dysbiosis and leaky gut contribute to the inflammatory process.[2] In addition, there is an association between dysbiosis and leaky gut and the resulting inflammation that is implicated in colorectal cancer.[3]

Doctors often break the immune system into two components: the innate immune system and the acquired or adaptive immune system. However, these two systems work in a complementary fashion to protect the body.

The innate immune system refers to the immunity you have at birth, and it lasts a lifetime. The innate immune system is the first responder to infectious organisms and rapid, nonspecific trauma. This includes protective barriers like the skin and mucous membranes, physiological factors (temperature/fever), pH and chemical factors, and several immune cells (*phagocytes*) that engulf microbes and remove waste products. Innate immunity has no memory or recognition of an infectious agent.

The acquired immune system plays an important role when innate immunity is not sufficient to eliminate a risk. Acquired immunity has the ability to recognize the foreign substances and the body's own tissues. Specialized cells, such as T cells, are involved in recognizing and destroying harmful microbes. Also, B cells can recognize foreign invaders and produce memory cells that will recognize intruders and maintain antibodies for a future response. For example, if you recently had a virus and were exposed to it again, those antibodies would kick in to protect you from getting sick again. Following is a brief summary of the many key players of the immune system.

Skin

Your skin is the first line of protection against infectious agents, cancer, and toxins. It is your largest organ and acts as an external barrier to pathogens. However, the skin also contains several immune cells. For example, the outer layer of the skin (*epidermis*) contains *keratinocytes,* which have receptors (toll-like receptors) that sense disease-causing microbes and trigger an immune response. The keratinocytes also contain *macrophages* that respond to infection and inflammation. In addition, there are several other immune cells of the skin that respond to inflammation and infection.

What is also interesting is that, like your gut, your skin harbors its own microbiome and contains millions of bacteria, fungi, and viruses.[4] The skin microbiome is acquired at birth from the vaginal canal or the skin with cesarean section. There is further colonization of the microbiota from breastfeeding. Dermatology research has shown that common skin conditions like acne and eczema are associated with changes in the microbiota of the skin. It has been well documented that an imbalance in the gut microbiome predisposes you to common skin conditions such as eczema, psoriasis, and rosacea.

There is ongoing research for both the topical and oral treatment of common skin conditions with probiotics. I believe that this category of treatment will become mainstream in the future. For now, holistic doctors like myself are already using oral prebiotics and probiotics to treat skin conditions, and increasingly using topical products as well.

Digestive Factors

There are several digestive factors that play a role in immunity. First, your saliva not only helps to break down carbohydrates and fats with enzymes but also works to produce antibodies such as IgA and IgG that help your immune system neutralize microbes. Next, your stomach acid (hydrochloric acid or HCL) liquefies food and breaks down proteins into amino acids. The HCL also lowers the stomach pH environment, which kills microorganisms directly and prevents the growth of microbes in the stomach and intestines.

White Blood Cells

You are probably familiar with the white blood cells that fight off infectious intruders, such as viruses, bacteria, and other microbes. There are different types of white blood cells that have designated functions for protecting your body. Your white blood cells require nutrients like zinc and vitamin C to function properly. Problems with malabsorption and nutrient deficiencies can lead to immune dysfunction.

Lymph Nodes

Lymph nodes are found in chains in various parts of the body, such as the groin, abdomen, chest, armpits, and neck. Lymphatic fluid contains *lymphocytes,* types of white blood cells, as well as other immune cells to fight infection. Lymphatic vessels transport the lymph fluid and return it to the venous system. The lymph nodes filter microbes, cancer cells, and toxins as well as act as sensors for foreign invaders.

Spleen

The spleen is a large organ located under the left ribs. It is part of the lymphatic system and filters and stores blood as well as produces white blood cells and antibodies to fight infection. Research has demonstrated that the gut microbiome interacts with the spleen.

Tonsils and Adenoids

Tonsils are collections of lymphatic tissue found in different parts of the throat. The adenoids are one type of tonsil, located high in the throat, that cannot be seen without the use of special instruments. These lymphatic organs trap microbes such as bacteria from food. Also, the tonsils produce antibodies to fight infections. Moreover, the microbiota of the mouth and throat (including the tonsils) contains more than 700 different bacterial species.[5] Research has shown that probiotic supplementation was helpful in the treatment of acute and chronic upper respiratory tract infections,[6] including the treatment of tonsillitis when used in conjunction with antibiotics.[7]

Thymus

Located behind the breastbone in the upper chest, the thymus gland functions to mature white blood cells known as *T lymphocytes*. Recent research has found a "gut-thymus axis" and the connection between intestinal microbiota and development of T cells.[8] Metabolites from the gut microbiome travel to and influence the thymus tissue.[9] Research is ongoing as how probiotics may benefit thymic activity.

Bone Marrow

Bone marrow refers to the spongy tissue found in the center of some bones, such as the hips and breastbone. It produces various types of cells including white blood cells. There have been recent publications demonstrating that the microbiota communicates with the bone marrow and influences the production of blood cells.[10]

Appendix

This organ is composed of lymphoid tissue and is located in the right lower quadrant of the abdomen where the intestine transitions to the colon. The appendix projects off the cecum, a part of the large intestine. It is a myth that the appendix serves no function, because it prevents infection by storing good bacteria and producing antibodies.[11]

Lymphoid Tissue and the Gut

People are surprised to find that the small intestine holds the largest mass of lymphoid tissue involved in immunity. This tissue supports immune responses and produces B and T lymphocytes, macrophages, antigen-presenting cells, and other specialist immune cells. This grouping of lymphoid tissue is also known as the gut-associated lymphoid tissues (GALT) or Peyer's patches.

Another immune system component is the intestine-draining mesenteric lymph nodes (MLN). The MLN are drainage sites for the small and large intestines and prevent intestinal bacteria from penetrating into systemic circulation. The MLN are also involved in T cell activation. Abnormalities in the microbiota of mesenteric lymph nodes are more common in people with ulcerative colitis.

These two components of the immune system in the small intestine fight infection and maintain a healthy gut barrier. According to *Mucosal Immunology*, "the intestine contains the greatest number and diversity of immune compartments and immune cells in the body."[12] Therefore, if you have a weak immune system or a dysregulated immune system (for example, you have autoimmune diseases or allergies), you should seek to improve the health of your gut.

HORMONE BALANCE

There has been a paradigm shift in the understanding of hormones produced and managed by the body. This shift in thinking involves the small intestine and specialized cells known as *enteroendocrine cells* (EE cells). *Frontiers in Physiology* reported that EE cells secrete hormones and make up the largest organ in the body, even though they account for less than 1 percent of the total gut epithelial cells.[13] These hormones, which influence many metabolic processes such as appetite, metabolism, and blood sugar regulation, include GLP-1, PYY, GIP, 5-HT, and CCK. The journal also reported that "the gut microbiome influences EE cell hormone release."

Chronic inflammation from dysbiosis and leaky gut sets the stage for hormone imbalance. There is a known two-way interaction between steroid hormones (e.g., estrogens, progesterone, testosterone, cortisol) and gut microbiota. *Frontiers in Microbiology* reported: "Hormones can have an impact on the composition and metabolism of the microbiota. In turn, the gut microbiome is highly involved in hormone homeostasis through a number of possible mechanisms."[14] It also noted that dysbiosis (which goes hand in hand with leaky gut) creates inflammation that negatively affects the enzyme metabolism of hormones in the gut and ultimately in the bloodstream. The term *endobolome* is now used to describe the interaction of the gut microbiota genes and the metabolism of steroid hormones and endocrine-disrupting chemicals (EDCs).[15]

A state of dysbiosis and diminished diversity of the microbiota can have a negative effect on the endobolome. An imbalance in the gut microbiota changes enzyme activity, which in turn prevents the efficient metabolism or breakdown of hormones. Since the endobolome affects the metabolism of hormones, it can result in hormone imbalance, including high levels of certain sex steroids or EDCs that increase the risk of sex-hormone-related cancers.[16]

Research with men and postmenopausal women has found that the urinary level of estrogen (both sexes have this hormone) is strongly associated with the number and diversity of stool microbiota. And studies with men have shown that gut microbial diversity affects testosterone levels. In addition, recent research reveals that gut permeability (leaky gut) increases during the menopausal transition in women.[17]

One area of important research involves the gut microbiome and women's hormonal disorders, including breast, endometrial, and ovarian cancers.[18] The estrobolome refers to the gut bacteria genes that are involved in estrogen metabolism. The research involves the microbiota and enzymatic reactions that reactivate certain estrogens to be recirculated in the body, instead of being broken down and excreted. As a result, there are higher blood levels of active estrogens, which may activate estrogen-positive cancers.

Another example of the gut-hormone link involves the most common cause of hypothyroidism (low thyroid), an autoimmune condition known as Hashimoto's thyroiditis (HT). HT is an autoimmune disease in which the immune system attacks thyroid gland tissue and makes one susceptible to the underproduction of thyroid hormones. According to research published in *Frontiers in Immunology,* "There is a lot of evidence that the intestinal dysbiosis, bacterial overgrowth, and increased intestinal permeability (leaky gut) favor HT development, and a Thyroid-Gut Axis has been proposed which seems to impact our entire metabolism."[19]

One last example of the gut-hormone link is melatonin. Known as the sleep hormone, melatonin is secreted by the pineal gland in the brain at nighttime to induce the sleep cycle. Researchers have now shown a relationship between the gut microbiota and melatonin production.[20] Interestingly, gut microbiota synthesize melatonin and possibly more than what is produced by the pineal gland. Studies show that dysbiosis reduces gut and pineal levels and that probiotics can increase systemic levels of melatonin. Moreover, melatonin itself may improve the functioning of microbiota and have positive effects on certain health conditions.

BLOOD SUGAR REGULATION

There is ongoing research connecting leaky gut and the risk of diabetes. For example, research in *Diabetes & Metabolism* found that biomarkers of leaky gut were significantly higher in people with type 2 diabetes.[21]

Recent research reveals that gut microbiota helps regulate blood sugar and insulin sensitivity. People with type 2 diabetes have been shown to have significant changes in their gut microbiota and their metabolites. An imbalance of the gut microbiota plays a role in the initiation and progression of type 2 diabetes by affecting the regulation of glucose and insulin sensitivity. Type 2 diabetes is mainly a condition of insulin resistance, wherein the cell receptors are resistant to the transportation of glucose into the cells. *Mediators of Inflammation* reported that: "Symptoms of diabetic patients can be improved by modifying gut microbiota."[22] They recommend consuming foods that act as prebiotics, exercising to improve gut microbiota, and taking probiotics as a source of friendly flora to improve glucose metabolism. Interestingly, the common type 2 diabetic medication known as Metformin appears to favorably alter the gut microbiota involved in glucose metabolism.

There is also research showing that dysbiosis is associated with the onset of type 1 diabetes, an autoimmune condition in which the immune system attacks and damages the insulin-producing cells of the pancreas. According to an article in *Frontiers in Endocrinology*, "A large body of evidence suggested that defective profile of intestinal microbiome may influence the pathogenesis of T1 D by affecting immune homeostasis and/or gut permeability."[23] Essentially, dysbiosis and leaky gut may cause type 1 diabetes by affecting the immune system in a damaging way.

METABOLISM AND WEIGHT

The effects of gut health also extend to metabolism and weight. According to research in *Frontiers in Endocrinology*, people who are "overweight" or "obese" have significant changes in their gut microbiota, which interferes with normal glucose and insulin metabolism.[24]

Researchers have recognized for years that the ratio and types of gut flora affect metabolism. For example, the microbiota play an important role in producing metabolites that act as hormones to regulate insulin sensitivity, glucose tolerance, fat storage, and appetite. *Frontiers in Physiology* reported that the small intestine cells make and secrete hormones that regulate appetite, fat deposition, and insulin sensitivity. These hormones include GLP-1, PYY, GIP, 5-HT, and CCK.[25]

In addition, some bacterial species such as *Lactobacillus* can promote weight loss while others promote weight gain. This effect seems to be related to the interactions between the gut microbiota, immune system, and gut intestinal function. While researchers are working on finding more specific protocols to change gut flora to help metabolism and weight, it makes sense if you are struggling with this issue to follow the protocols in this book to create a gut ecology favorable to good metabolism.

BRAIN AND NERVOUS SYSTEM

Researchers have proven a direct connection between the gut microbiome and intestinal permeability and the brain and nervous system, which has led to our knowledge of a *gut-brain axis* and *gut-brain-microbiota axis*. There is emerging evidence that disruptions in gut health, such as the leaky gut, adversely affect brain function. This gut-brain relationship has been most well studied in people with celiac disease and autism spectrum disorder (ASD).[26] However, among my patients, I regularly see improvements in all types of cognitive issues with natural healing gut protocols.

Leaky gut and dysbiosis have negative impacts on the brain. When the intestinal blood barrier is compromised, it has the potential to affect various organ systems of the body adversely.[27] The brain has a design similar to the small intestine in that it has a barrier known as the blood-brain barrier (BBB). A leaky gut may be an underlying cause for disruptions in the BBB.[28] The systemic inflammatory response by the immune system to the leaky gut may lead to disruptive effects on the BBB. Some refer to the increased permeability of the BBB as a "leaky brain." A breakdown in the BBB has been observed in patients with major psychiatric illnesses.[29] The neurological conditions associated with a "leaky brain" include autism spectrum disorder (ASD), dementia, Alzheimer's disease, depression, schizophrenia, multiple sclerosis, brain trauma, edema, brain cancers, amyotrophic lateral sclerosis (ALS), and meningitis.

Interestingly, an article in *Food Science and Human Wellness* stated that nerves traveling from the brain (vagus nerves) connect with the microbiome![30] Therefore, brain activity directly influences the microbiome. As a result, stress responses by the brain may cause dysbiosis in the gut. Oppositely, the article stated that an inflamed gut with dysbiosis can influence brain activity by altering neurotransmitter (brain chemical) balance. Several neurotransmitters, such as serotonin, acetylcholine, histamine, GABA, and glutamate, can affect gut health and activity. An unhealthy gut is known to cause the release of the stress hormone in the brain known as adrenocorticotropic hormone (ACTH), which causes the adrenal glands to release stress hormones.

While we know the foods we eat affect the health of our microbiota, there is also research demonstrating that a high-stress lifestyle contributes to dysbiosis. Stress and depression can change gut bacteria's composition due to changes in stress hormones, inflammation, and nervous system changes.[31] As a result of unfavorable changes in gut microbiota from stress and mood problems, it further contributes to the cycle of additional problems with adapting to stress and improving one's mood. And lastly, gut dysbiosis is associated with severe mental illness and is a research priority.[32]

MUSCLES, JOINTS, AND BONES

The connection between our gut bacteria and intestinal health extends to our muscles, joints, and bones. An increase in inflammation from leaky gut and dysbiosis wreaks havoc on the muscles and joints of the body. There has been a lot of research on this subject, especially concerning autoimmune diseases that affect the musculoskeletal system. The term *gut-joint axis* describes the connection between the two systems.

There could be detrimental effects in genetically predisposed people who are exposed to environmental factors that negatively affect the microbiome gut and, therefore, the immune system.[33] Clinical reports suggest that leaky gut syndrome contributes to autoimmune diseases of the joints such as rheumatoid arthritis.[34]

There have been other studies demonstrating alterations in gut microbiota as well as leaky gut and an association with the auto-immune condition known as psoriatic arthritis.

Of great interest is the association between leaky gut and osteoarthritis (OA). OA is the most common joint condition in humans. A review of studies, mainly animal but some human, suggested that leaky gut and dysbiosis create an environment of joint inflammation and progression of OA disease. Alterations in the gut microbiome due to dysbiosis promotes inflammation in the joints, including OA.[35] This OA inflammatory response can be decreased with dietary changes, prebiotics, and probiotics.

Your bones are also connected to your gut in the *gut-bone axis*. An imbalance in the gut can contribute to bone mass loss through chronic inflammation as well as nutrient deficiencies. The *Journal of Leukocyte Biology* reported that the gut microbiota are emerging as an important modulator of bone metabolism.[36] The journal noted that prebiotics and probiotics improved calcium absorption and enhanced bone mineralization as well as increased availability of magnesium and phosphorous. In addition, short chain fatty acids produced by gut bacteria fermentation on carbohydrates modulates osteoclasts and osteoblast, cells involved in bone turnover. In one study, researchers found that menopausal women had greater degrees of leaky gut.[37] The increased gut permeability was also associated with increased markers of inflammation and lower bone mineral density.

Research is now demonstrating that probiotics may help improve bone density. A study published in the *Journal of Internal Medicine* found that probiotic supplementation in women between the ages of 75 and 80 resulted in increased bone density compared to those taking a placebo.[38] The same researchers noted that the gut microbiome modulates the immune system and the bone-metabolizing cells known as osteoclasts.

CARDIOVASCULAR HEALTH

The relationship between cardiovascular health and the gut is known as the *gut-heart axis*. According to researchers from the medical journal *Open Heart*, "The intestinal microbiome plays a role in the pathogenesis of atherosclerosis and heart failure."[39] The same authors noted that people with inflammatory bowel disease have permeability problems with the small intestine (leaky gut) and a much higher risk of coronary heart disease. The increased absorption in the bloodstream of bacterial toxins from leaky gut leads to a chronic inflammatory state and increased risk of cardiovascular disease.

Research demonstrates that the gut microbiota help to metabolize lipids and exhibit a protective effect on the development of plaque in the arteries (atherosclerosis). Some researchers suggest that measuring certain gut microbiota should be considered as diagnostic markers for people with coronary artery disease.[40]

ENERGY PRODUCTION

Your cells require many different nutrients to produce energy. A leaky gut can impair the proper nutrient absorption necessary for cellular energy. The bacterial toxins absorbed with leaky gut also contribute to inflammation and reduced energy production.

Gut microbiota promotes energy production by playing a role in glucose metabolism and producing short-chain fatty acids and B vitamins used to produce energy. Research has revealed that there is a two-way communication between the microbiota and the energy-producing factors in cells known as mitochondria.[41] The metabolites of the microbiota, such as short-chain fatty acids and other compounds, stimulate energy production and help control inflammation that occurs with the mitochondria. On the other end, mitochondria have a regulating effect on the gut microbiota by modulating the intestinal barrier and mucosal immune response.

A severe form of longstanding fatigue is known as chronic fatigue syndrome (CFS), also referred to as myalgic encephalomyelitis (ME). Studies have shown that people with this condition have a decrease in the microbiome of firmicutes and increased bacteroidetes. *Molecular Psychiatry* reported that gut dysbiosis is associated with chronic fatigue.[42]

There are many organs and biochemical pathways that affect energy production. Since a leaky gut affects all the organs of the body, it makes sense that if you want to have optimal energy production, it is critical to address a leaky gut. The combination of prebiotics and probiotics have been shown to improve the production of short-chain fatty acids used for energy production.

URINARY HEALTH

As with other systems of the body, a connection exists between the gut and urinary organs (kidney and bladder).[43] There is evidence that dysbiosis plays a direct role in urinary tract infections. Research has shown that an abundance of *E. Coli* bacteria in the gut was associated with future urinary tract infections with *E. Coli*. Repeat urinary tract infections may be due to an overabundance of infectious agents in the gut that cause urinary tract infections and act as a reservoir for infection. We now recognize that gut dysbiosis should be considered a target of treatment for those with recurring urinary tract infections. In addition, gut dysbiosis can play an indirect role in kidney disorders such as hypertension, chronic kidney disease, and urinary stones.

The urinary tract has its own microbiome. It was thought that the urinary tract was sterile; however, there is urinary microbiota in the bladder and urinary tract. Researchers are now investigating the role of a healthy urinary microbiome and the *gut-urinary axis* in preventing urinary tract infections.

DENTAL HEALTH

There is also a *gut-gum axis*, which refers to inflammation and dysbiosis in the gums (periodontitis and gingivitis) that then allow microbes to transfer through saliva to the gut.[44] It includes microbes transferring from the gut to the gums. According to the *Journal of Oral Microbiology*, the bacteria *Porphyromonas gingivalis* creates dysbiosis in the microbiota of the gums, and then transfer by saliva to the gut and play a role in gut dysbiosis.[45]

EYE HEALTH

There is new evidence for the *gut-eye axis*, whereby gut dysbiosis may be an important factor that influences the triggering and progression of several eye diseases, including uveitis, dry eye, macular degeneration, and glaucoma.[46] Eye inflammation seems to be influenced by dysbiosis of the gut flora.[47] This includes conditions such as age-related macular degeneration, diabetic retinopathy, and retinitis pigmentosa.

The gut-eye axis is an emerging field of study that could provide more fundamental and root-cause therapies for people with eye conditions. The surface of the eye contains its own microbiome, which responds to disease-causing bacteria as part of an immune response. Imbalances in the eye microbiome are thought to predispose us to several eye diseases, including blepharitis, conjunctivitis, dry eye syndrome, and others.

REPRODUCTIVE HEALTH

The female reproductive tract, which refers to the vulva, cervix, endometrium, fallopian tubes, and ovaries, has its own unique microbiome. The content of the microbiome changes depending on the stage of life and phase of the menstrual cycle. This microbiome is important in preventing conditions such as preterm birth and reproductive tract infections. Much of the research on the female reproductive tract involves the vaginal microbiome. A healthy vaginal microbiome is necessary to produce compounds such as hydrogen peroxide and other agents that fight local infection. *Lactobacillus* are the dominate flora in the vaginal microbiome and are important for maintaining a low vaginal pH.[48] Conditions such as bacterial vaginosis are characterized by a large drop in the total number of *Lactobacillus*.

The gut and female genital tract are in constant communication with one another.[49] In addition, the dominant *Lactobacillus* species of the vaginal tract is thought to originate from the gut. The microbiota of the gut and vagina have a close interaction, so problems with the gut microbiome, which metabolizes estrogen, can result in conditions related to the female reproductive tract.

The male reproductive tract also has a microbiome. Leaky gut can result in immune system activation that can negatively influence the testicles and male reproduction.[50] Moreover, the testicles have been found to have their own microbiome. Even semen has its own microbiome, with some research suggesting that good-quality sperm have different microbiota than low-quality semen. Supplementation with probiotics has been shown to improve sperm count and motility for infertile men.[51]

SKIN HEALTH

The skin is one of the largest organs of the body, and the gut microbiome plays a role in inflammatory skin diseases.[52] There is a "gut-skin axis" that must be addressed when dealing with chronic skin conditions. Studies have revealed that children with eczema have significantly lower levels of the friendly flora *Bifidobacterium* and higher levels of the bacteria staphylococcus.[53] Research published in the *The Quarterly Journal of Medicine* as far back as 1985 reported leaky gut in people with eczema and psoriasis.[54]

And as I mentioned earlier in this chapter, the skin has its own microbiome that is separate from the gut. However, the gut-skin axis can influence the skin and its microbiome positively or negatively.

DETOXIFICATION

Your body is exposed to numerous environmental chemicals that can be detrimental to your health. The GI tract is where most environmental toxins enter the body (food, water, drugs). While we think of the liver as the major organ of detoxification, researchers have found that the gut microbiota are just as potent in the breakdown of toxins.[55] Environmental toxins can be inactivated by the gut microbiome as well as metabolized and broken down. Research has also shown that the gut microbiota can be adversely affected by environmental pollutants.[56]

Preliminary studies are now suggesting that probiotics have beneficial effects on heavy metals (arsenic, cadmium, lead, mercury, and others) by promoting detoxification and excretion.[57] Nutrition-oriented practitioners are now using prebiotics and probiotics to help with detoxification.

GUT HEALTH

There is an obvious connection between leaky gut and digestive diseases. The most well-studied link includes inflammatory bowel disease (Crohn's disease and ulcerative colitis), celiac disease, and non-celiac gluten sensitivity. Increased gastrointestinal permeability (leaky gut) also occurs in irritable bowel syndrome (IBS) research.[58] Many studies have demonstrated that dysbiosis is very common with IBS.

Even food sensitivities and food allergies can be related to leaky gut. This condition allows for undigested food particles to enter the bloodstream, which can result in food allergies.[59]

○ ○ ◉ ○ ○

As you have read, there is a connection between the health of your gut and the functioning of the organs in your body. You can see how holistic medicine helps whole-body health by treating digestive imbalances.

Chapter 3

WHAT CAUSES LEAKY GUT?

Paul, a 56-year-old store owner, had been suffering from abdominal pains and loose stool for several years. Colonoscopy testing did not show any abnormalities. In talking with him, I found out he had been taking aspirin as a preventative medication for heart disease and stroke. In analyzing his cardiovascular risk, I told him that he not only did not need aspirin, but also that it is a well-known cause of ulcers and leaky gut. He discontinued the aspirin, followed my diet and supplement advice, and his digestive symptoms cleared completely within three weeks.

There are several causes of leaky gut and dysbiosis. Many of these causes are related to diet, lifestyle choices, and medications. Fortunately, most of these causes can be resolved through diet and lifestyle changes as well as nutritional and holistic therapies that heal the gut. In this chapter we'll take a look at the most common reasons why people develop leaky gut—from common medications and infections to genetics, exercise, and even aging—and how to determine if you have it.

The following causes are addressed in this chapter, in alphabetical order:

- aging
- alcohol
- chemotherapy and radiation
- chronic illnesses
- disrupted nerve and blood flow to the gut
- dust mite allergens
- dysbiosis
- excessive exercise
- genetics
- gluten allergy/sensitivity and food sensitivities
- hormone and neurotransmitter imbalance
- infections
- medications
- nonalcoholic fatty liver disease (NAFLD or MASLD)
- nutritional deficiencies
- poor diet (industrialized Western diet)
- psychological stress
- smoking
- weight issues and insulin resistance
- xenobiotics—chemicals foreign to the body

AGING

The microbiota is most susceptible to instability during infancy and old age. As we age, there is increased susceptibility to gut dysbiosis and gut pathogens, inflammation, more medication use, decreased immunity, and leaky gut.[1] *Genes & Immunity* acknowledged that alterations in the gut microbiome is one of the concerns with aging, immune system breakdown disorders, and frailty. An aging microbiota may affect general health, especially the gut-brain axis.[2] There is ongoing research to see if improving the gut microbiota can help with healthy aging.

ALCOHOL

Alcohol is absorbed in the small intestine. Many studies have shown that alcohol causes dysbiosis where good bacteria is reduced, and potentially harmful bacteria is increased. Alcohol causes leaky gut by disrupting and damaging transcellular and paracellular pathways involved in small intestine absorption (see the Sensational Small Intestine section on page 13 for a review).[3]

Alcohol harms the small intestine epithelial cells. It causes cell death, converts into acetaldehyde that damages cell DNA, increases damaging free radicals, and causes gut inflammation. Alcohol also depletes the body of gut-healing nutrients such as vitamin A and D and the mineral zinc, which are discussed later in the book.

CHEMOTHERAPY AND RADIATION

Researchers in the cancer journal *Acta Oncologica* reported that: "Gastrointestinal (GI) symptoms are the most common of all consequences of cancer treatment and have the greatest impact on daily activity."[4] Research published in *Frontiers in Behavioral Neuroscience* has shown that the brain and gut are the two organs that are most vulnerable to the toxicities of chemotherapy.[5] The same paper noted that chemotherapy causes chemotherapy-induced gut toxicity (CIGT) damage. Chemotherapy impairs the intestinal barrier by causing defects in the tight junction integrity, and it alters the microbiota, which also contributes to leaky gut.

In addition, chemotherapy damages the nerves between the layers of the muscles in the gastrointestinal tract, known as the *myenteric plexus,* which are involved in peristalsis (contraction of intestines that propels food and waste products). Lastly, chemotherapy toxicity causes brain changes that affect signaling to the gut (gut-brain axis).

Radiation therapy has also been shown to cause gut problems. According to *Nutrients*, "There is overwhelming evidence to show that the gut microbiome is significantly altered by radiation."[6] This radiation-induced microbiome change is problematic in patients receiving radiation therapy to the abdominal region. Radiation therapy to the abdominal area also causes small intestinal bacterial overgrowth (SIBO) in 25 percent of patients. This overgrowth of bacteria in the small intestine leads to malabsorption and sets the stage for a leaky gut. On the other hand, *Radiation Oncology* reported that the state of the gut microbiome can influence the effectiveness of radiation therapy, degree of digestive toxicity and damage from cancer therapy, and cancer therapy in general.[7] A meta-analysis of six studies involving 917 participants with pelvic or abdominal cancers found that probiotic supplementation was beneficial to prevent diarrhea caused by radiation therapy.[8]

CHRONIC ILLNESSES

In the earlier Chemotherapy and Radiation section on page 47, I discussed how people undergoing chemotherapy and radiation therapies are prone to disrupting their microbiota and leaky gut. However, it's the nature of chronic illnesses that they often involve pain, reduced activity, high stress, nutritional deficiencies, and gut-damaging medications—all of which make you more susceptible to leaky gut. If you have a chronic illness, you are more vulnerable to a leaky gut. And as I mentioned earlier, since your gut health affects your whole body, addressing leaky gut can help you manage or treat a chronic illness. In the section on Hormone and Neurotransmitter Imbalance on page 52, you will see further how the stress of chronic illness affects gut health.

DISRUPTED NERVE AND BLOOD FLOW TO THE GUT

There is a higher-than-normal amount of blood flow to the gastrointestinal tract organs, with 25 percent of the cardiac (heart) output going to this region. The superior mesenteric artery feeds blood supply to the small intestine, and there are control mechanisms for ensuring blood flow to the intestines. Blood flow includes metabolic control, where special sensors assess metabolites such as oxygen, carbon dioxide, and others. When nutrients like oxygen are low (or carbon dioxide is high), the local blood vessels dilate for improved blood flow. The stretching of the intestinal muscles with food results in blood vessel relaxation and dilation, and messages from the nervous system also increase or decrease blood flow.

Intestinal cell health depends on blood and nerve flow to bring in oxygen and nutrients for healthy cell regeneration (intestinal stem cell activity is also essential). A holistic view of gut health would include any obstacle to small intestine blood flow. Examples that can impede blood flow and nervous system messaging include a poor diet, deficient digestive juices and enzymes, reduced beneficial flora, gut infections, musculoskeletal problems including neck and back disorders, any chronic pain, subluxations, and poor stress coping mechanisms. Musculoskeletal treatments such as chiropractic, osteopathic manipulation, massage, acupuncture, and physical therapy can help digestive health by improving nerve and blood flow.

One of the most common disrupters of blood flow is mental stress. Extended periods of mental stress result in a reduction of blood flow to digestive organs, which disrupts the regenerative capacity of the intestinal mucosa and an increase in the production of toxic metabolites.[9]

See also the section in this chapter: Psychological Stress on page 57.

DUST MITE ALLERGENS

Environmental allergens may be linked to leaky gut, and a common allergen that has been studied is dust mites. In the journal *Gut*, a study of people with a house dust-mite allergy found that it contributed to leaky gut, as it increased intestinal permeability.[10] Your doctor can test you for dust-mite allergies. Common symptoms include sneezing, runny nose, and aggravation of asthma symptoms. If you know you have a dust mite allergy, then using materials in your home such as sheets, pillows, blinds, and others that can be washed with warm water is helpful. In addition, allergists can provide dust mite desensitization treatment.

DYSBIOSIS

Many of the root causes you read about in this section of the book contribute to dysbiosis, which refers to the overgrowth of harmful microbes and the depletion of healthy microbes in the gut. There is an avalanche of research revealing how dysbiosis contributes to leaky gut. *Frontiers in Immunology* reported that dysbiosis causes mucosal barrier dysfunction, increased inflammation, and leaky gut.[11] Also, SIBO (small intestine bacterial overgrowth) is an example where colonic bacteria migrate to the small intestine and create dysbiosis. As a result of the inflammation and gut-altering effects, leaky gut occurs.

EXCESSIVE EXERCISE

Low- to moderate-intensity exercise has positive effects on gut health and contributes to a healthy intestinal mucosa.[12] A balanced exercise intensity has been shown to improve gut barrier health and immune activity in the gut and increase friendly flora. On the other hand, excessive or too strenuous exercise can lead to a leaky gut.[13] One of the reasons for this is that the sympathetic nervous system responds to exercise by reducing blood flow to the digestive organs and increasing blood flow to the working muscles. The lack of blood flow leads to unfavorable changes in the gut mucus, immune cells, and tight junctions that prevent undesirable particles and organisms from being absorbed. In addition, decreased nerve activity to the intestine can affect absorption. The two biggest determinants of exercise causing leaky gut are intensity of the exercise and volume of training. Researchers have found that ≥ 70 percent of maximum working capacity and a volume of more than one hour can cause leaky gut. However, there are other factors involved, such as temperature, food consumed during the training process, attitude, fluid restriction, degree of trainability, and the times of day that training occur.

GENETICS

Genetics can also play a role in your predisposition to leaky gut. Researchers reported in *Gut* that genetic mutations associated with Crohn's disease have been identified.[14] People with Crohn's disease and first-degree relatives are more likely to have leaky gut. More research is needed to assess the role of genetics and predisposition to leaky gut; however, the good news is that we can often offset the expression of our genes through a healthy diet and lifestyle, and the use of specific supplementation.

GLUTEN ALLERGY/SENSITIVITY AND FOOD SENSITIVITIES

Undiagnosed gluten allergy (celiac disease) has been a significant cause of leaky gut and damaged small intestine. Many people who do not have celiac disease have what is known as non-celiac gluten sensitivity. People sensitive to gluten can also experience unhealthy changes to their small intestine lining. And along these same lines, integrative doctors have found that food sensitivities or intolerances contribute to leaky gut. Food intolerance affects 15 to 20 percent of the population.[15] We should also consider that a leaky gut can cause food sensitivities. An elimination diet or blood food allergy/intolerance testing is available through integrative doctors for further assessment.

HORMONE AND NEUROTRANSMITTER IMBALANCE

There is a direct interaction between the body's hormones, neurotransmitters, and the gut. The gut-brain-microbiota axis plays a role in the communication systems of the body. More specifically, the body responds to stress through the hypothalamic-pituitary-adrenal (HPA) axis, and leaky gut and dysbiosis can activate the HPA axis.[16] This communication network uses hormones and neurotransmitters to respond to various stresses—physical, mental, and emotional. The brain takes information from the outside world though our senses, and it is deciphered by various areas of the brain, and then messaging from the hypothalamus goes to the pituitary gland, and then to the adrenal glands, which are the stress-hormone-producing glands. Bacteria metabolites (LPS) can be absorbed through the gut due to leaky gut and affect the development and behavior of the brain. Also, prebiotics and probiotics can help modulate the inflammation that leads to activation of the HPA Axis. Essentially, leaky gut and dysbiosis can be related to neurotransmitter and hormone imbalances due to the dynamic interrelationship between these body systems.

INFECTIONS

Undiagnosed and untreated infections in the gut (fungal, bacterial, viral, or parasitic) lead to gut wall inflammation. Any type of gut infection, whether acute or chronic—and especially chronic—can lead to gut wall inflammation and leaky gut.

One example of a gut bacterial infection that can cause leaky gut is *Helicobacter pylori*, also referred to as *H. pylori*. These bacteria can be acquired through sharing drinking cups, utensils, and kissing. For some people it causes gastritis, resulting in stomach pain, and sometimes nausea and bloating.

Gut Pathogens reported that refined sugars are food sources for disease-causing microbes in the intestines: "By consuming too much refined sugar, the populations of health-promoting bacteria in the digestive system are reduced, and the populations of pathogenic bacteria and fungi like *Candida albicans* (C. albicans) flourished, which can result in leaky gut."[17] The use of antibiotics to treat infections can also lead to fungal overgrowth.

Infections in the gut can become chronic, according to *Microbiological Research*: "C. albicans can grow, proliferate, and coexist with the host for a long time."[18] Like other microbes, *C. albicans* and other fungi protect themselves against the immune system by creating a biofilm—a collection of microorganisms that stick to a surface and one another. Biofilms make it more difficult for the immune system to remove them. In addition, C. albicans is a normal part of the gut flora but can colonize the intestine excessively when antibiotics are used.[19] Excess C. albicans results in a disruption of the intestinal mucosa barrier.

According to the Centers for Disease Control, parasitic infections are not uncommon in the United States, "and in some cases, affect millions of people. Often, they can go unnoticed, with few symptoms."[20] And a recent article in *Signal Transduction and Targeted Therapy* discussed how COVID-19 attacks the digestive tract and likely contributes to gut permeability problems.[21]

As you can see, there are many ways that different microbes can infect your gut and make you susceptible to digestive problems and leaky gut. An integrative doctor can help you test for infectious agents of the digestive tract with stool and other lab assessments.

MEDICATIONS

According to *Frontiers in Pharmacology*, "Medication has recently emerged as one of the most influential determinants of the gut microbiota composition and activity."[22] It has been known for more than a decade that almost 70 percent of Americans take at least one prescription drug, and more than half take two. Of course, many people take over-the-counter drugs too.[23]

Also, those who take prescription medications take four medications on average. I will review some of the more well-studied medications that cause leaky gut. However, many medications may cause imbalances in the gut flora and contribute to a leaky gut. For example, a study published in *Nature* screened more than 1,000 marketed drugs and their effect on gut bacterial strains.[24] Researchers found that 24 percent of the drugs inhibited at least one strain. Many of the drugs functioned like antibiotics and reduced normal gut microbiota.

See also the section in this chapter: Chemotherapy and Radiation on page 47.

NSAIDs

Americans commonly use nonsteroidal anti-inflammatory drugs known as NSAIDs to treat pain and inflammation. Examples of NSAIDs include aspirin, ibuprofen, indomethacin, naproxen, diclofenac, and coxibs (e.g., celecoxib). According to an article in *Frontiers in Pharmacology*, short- and long-term use of NSAIDs can result in upper and lower digestive tract damage.[25] The article also noted that small intestine permeability (leaky gut) is present in 50 to 70 percent of long-term NSAID users! *Comprehensive Toxicology* reported that up to 20 percent of people who use NSAIDs regularly develop ulcers and 3 percent develop bowel hemorrhage or perforation.[26]

The leaky gut effects of NSAIDs are concerning. If you are on long-term NSAID use, I strongly recommend seeking holistic methods to heal or control your pain. Several therapies can treat many of the root causes of pain, such as chiropractic, acupuncture, naturopathic medicine, laser therapy, physical therapy, and natural anti-pain and anti-inflammatory supplements. In addition, addressing your leaky gut can effectively treat many types of non-injury-related pain conditions, as outlined in this book.

PPIs

Proton pump inhibitors (PPIs) are used to prevent and treat acid reflux, and these medications have been shown to affect the gut microbiota negatively. Research has revealed that when PPIs are given along with NSAIDs, they can have detrimental effects on the small intestine through dysbiosis and leaky gut.[27] The acid suppression of PPIs also causes small intestine bacterial overgrowth (SIBO), which causes malabsorption. One other known risk of PPI use is the increased risk of *C. difficile* infection, which is overgrowth of the bacteria clostridium difficile, resulting in diarrhea, abdominal pain, and fever.

Antibiotics

Antibiotics can negatively disrupt the gut microbiota. While they do destroy harmful and infectious bacteria, unfortunately they can also destroy and alter good bacteria. Remember that gut flora function as guards of the intestinal tract, preventing and regulating the growth of disease-causing microbes. Research has shown that infants given antibiotics right after birth have changes to their microbiota. This sets the stage for a leaky gut from an early age.[28] There is also emerging research that antibiotic use and changes in gut flora are related to the risk of developing type 2 diabetes.[29]

NONALCOHOLIC FATTY LIVER DISEASE (NAFLD OR MASLD)

According to the National Institutes of Health, approximately 30 percent of American adults have liver disease unrelated to alcohol consumption, historically known as nonalcoholic fatty liver disease (NAFLD).[30] Recently, the term NAFLD has been changed to metabolic dysfunction-associated steatotic liver disease (MASLD). (I will use the term NAFLD, as most people are not familiar with the new term MASLD.) NAFLD is the most common type of liver disease in the Western world, which stems from a buildup of excess fat in the liver. People who are obese or have type 2 diabetes are at much higher risk for NAFLD.

Studies have revealed that leaky gut appears to be increased in people with NAFLD, due to an interaction between the gut and liver, known as the *gut-liver axis*.[31] The communication between these two organs is facilitated by the intestinal barrier. If a leaky gut occurs, then bacteria that are usually not absorbed in a healthy gut are taken from the intestines to the liver by the portal vein. As a result, the liver must deal with these bacterial toxins (known as endotoxins), creating an inflammatory response. People with NAFLD often have dysbiosis, another known cause of leaky gut.[32]

NUTRITIONAL DEFICIENCIES

As with any tissue in the body, the small intestine requires proper nutrients. Vitamins A and D are intricately involved in the healthy tight junctions of the small intestine.[33] Also, vitamin D deficiencies or low levels of vitamin D are quite common. Zinc is also a key nutrient for a healthy gut microbiota and intestinal lining.[34]

A smaller percentage of people have deficiencies in vitamin A and zinc. However, you may have suboptimal levels that impair your gut health. Research also shows that omega-3 fatty acids promote small intestine health, and so a deficiency can contribute to a leaky gut.[35] Later in this book, I discuss research on how the nutrients quercetin, glutamine, and others play pivotal roles in healing leaky gut.

POOR DIET (INDUSTRIALIZED WESTERN DIET)

An unhealthy diet sets the stage for leaky gut, and researchers agree that the industrialized Western diet is a recipe for illness. (This is also known as the Standard American Diet or SAD.) Before unhealthy foods are digested and absorbed, they meet the gut, creating inflammation and intestinal damage. A low-fiber diet and high sugar intake bathe intestinal lining.[36] While I will discuss much more about diet later in the book, the good news is that consuming gut-healthy foods can quickly improve intestinal and microbiome health.

PSYCHOLOGICAL STRESS

As discussed, researchers have shown a direct connection between the gut microbiome and intestinal permeability, with the brain and nervous system connection, also known as the *gut-brain axis* or *gut-brain-microbiota axis*. Given this link, stress and anxiety can have a direct impact on the gut. According to *Frontiers in Behavioral Neuroscience*, "Psychological and social factors can influence motility and digestive function."[37] Researchers have found that both acute and chronic stress can lead to changes in gut bacteria.[38] This includes the effects of stress and depression, which cause inflammation and the triggering of dysbiosis and leaky gut.

SMOKING

Smoking harms every organ of the body, and the gut is no exception. *Frontiers in Endocrinology* reported that "cigarette smoking plays a significant role in gut dysbiosis."[39] In addition, smoking causes the formation of free radicals, which damage the tissues of the body. It is also a vasoconstrictor that reduces blood flow to the gut. Research has shown that smoking damages the gut mucosa and impairs the immune system response in the gut.[40] To allow your gut to heal, it is vital to stop smoking.

WEIGHT ISSUES AND INSULIN RESISTANCE

According to the Centers for Disease Control, the number of U.S. adults who are "overweight" or "obese," is 73.6 percent.[41] Being overweight is a risk factor for leaky gut syndrome, especially if you also have a fatty liver.[42]

People with obesity have a lower percentage of the flora *Akkermancia muciniphila*, which is associated with healthy intestinal mucus and gut barrier.[43] Increasing this bacterium can improve insulin resistance, which is a factor for weight gain and diabetes risk.[44] People with obesity also have higher circulating levels of LPS, a marker of leaky gut.

Even young adults with insulin resistance are susceptible to leaky gut. A study published in *Diabetes, Metabolic Syndrome and Obesity: Targets and Therapy* found that leaky gut was associated with insulin resistance in young adults.[45] The same researchers noted that "abdominal obesity" is associated with leaky gut and dysbiosis, likely due to the consumption of the industrialized Western diet. ("Abdominal obesity" refers to having a high level of visceral fat, meaning a person has a high level of belly fat surrounding their organs.) Zonulin levels, a leaky gut marker, are typically higher in those of a higher weight.

If you are heavier than your preferred or ideal weight, it is particularly important to resolve leaky gut and dysbiosis. Many of my patients report they are able to lose weight more easily and that their elevated insulin and glucose levels drop when they follow my program. This is not surprising since the Mediterranean diet, and even more so with the reduced grain intake in my modified version, has been shown to help with weight and diabetes.

XENOBIOTICS—CHEMICALS FOREIGN TO THE BODY

There are more than 100,000 artificial chemicals in existence. According to the World Health Organization, nearly one in four of total global deaths are due to being exposed to an unhealthy environment.[46] Toxins can affect the body, including the gut, in many different negative ways. In a study conducted with mice that were designed to mimic the chemical exposure of Gulf War veterans, the researchers noted that Gulf War Illness included several disturbances in the body related to these chemicals.[47] Their study found that similar chemical exposure in mice resulted in significant dysbiosis and leaky gut. Moreover, endocrine-disrupting chemicals are known to adversely affect the gut microbiome.[48]

Toxics discussed how the gut microbiome metabolizes and helps to detoxify toxins such as arsenic, for example.[49] However, it reported that environmental toxins, such as toxic metals (e.g., lead and arsenic), pesticides, and others cause gut microbiome toxicity.[50] The widely used herbicide glyphosate, which is sprayed on many of our grains (wheat and corn) and fruit and vegetable crops, causes dysbiosis.[51] The United States has a much higher allowance for the acceptable daily intake of glyphosate compared to some countries in Europe and Canada.[52] In addition, researchers are finding a connection between wheat and gluten sensitivity and glyphosate levels in wheat.[53]

DO I HAVE LEAKY GUT OR DYSBIOSIS?

You may be wondering by now if you have leaky gut or dysbiosis. The fact is that many people with known chronic digestive problems have leaky gut. Yet there are all sorts of conditions that may be caused by an underlying problem with leaky gut or dysbiosis—and those issues may be the first sign of compromised gut health.

Here are a few symptoms and factors to consider when trying to determine if you have leaky gut or dysbiosis:

- Do you consume an unhealthy diet?
- Do you overconsume alcohol?

- Do you commonly have one or more of the following digestive symptoms: gas, bloating, abdominal distention, constipation, or diarrhea?

- Do you have a diagnosis of digestive illness, such as inflammatory bowel Disease, irritable Bowel syndrome (IBS), or small intestine bacterial overgrowth (SIBO)?

- Do you have bad breath?

- Do you have multiple food sensititivities?

- Do you have a chronic health condition or disease, whether physical (i.e., skin, brain, muscles/joints, etc.) or mental/emotional?

- Do you regularly or semi-regularly use medications that harm the gut and microbiome?

- Do you have chronic stress that is not resolving?

- Are you overtraining in sports?

- Have you been diagnosed with deficiencies of vitamins and minerals?

If you realize that you likely have leaky gut or dysbiosis then it is time to take action. You can consult with a functional or integrative medical professional who can guide you on the best courses of action. Feel free to talk to your medical provider about your concerns of leaky gut and SIBO. However, there is a high likelihood they will know little to nothing about the subject. You can also follow the recommendations in this book, assuming you have a healthcare professional to oversee your protocols.

CLINICAL MARKERS FOR LEAKY GUT

There are different ways clinicians can identify leaky gut. Besides the invasive assessment of intestinal tissue, some biomarkers can indicate a leaky gut. Your functional or integrative doctor may recommend certain labs to test for leaky gut. I should point out that there is no consensus on the best testing method for this condition. Currently available tests used by general practitioners include blood, stool, and urine. The following review does not encompass all the potential leaky gut testing options, some of which are invasive.

Zonulin

The intestinal cells release a family of proteins known as zonulin to respond to factors that threaten gut permeability, so their presence can serve as a biomarker. Zonulin activation appears to be a defense mechanism by the body to eradicate harmful microorganisms or toxins.[54] In other words, this is an intelligent system designed to protect the body. However, when the cause is unresolved, the leaky gut condition progresses, and more problems ensue.

Two of the most well-studied triggers of zonulin are substantial amounts of bacteria (such as bacterial overgrowth) and gluten (protein causing celiac disease and gluten sensitivity). It is thought that zonulin acts as a defense mechanism against microorganisms and gluten (which may also be recognized by the immune system as a foreign invader). When zonulin is released, it leads to the release of inflammatory chemicals (cytokines) that increase intestinal permeability. Measuring lab values of zonulin is one way to assess leaky gut status. An increased value is associated with increased intestinal permeability and tight junction dysfunction.

Research has shown that blood levels of zonulin are elevated in people with celiac disease and irritable bowel syndrome (IBS). In patients with IBS-D (diarrhea type), elevated levels of zonulin were similar to people with celiac disease. There are also labs that offer zonulin testing as part of stool analysis.

LPS

Lipopolysaccharides (LPS) refer to a component from the surface membrane of gram-negative bacteria. When LPS is absorbed into the bloodstream due to a leaky gut, it causes an inflammatory response. Adding insult to injury, research has also shown that the inflammatory effect of LPS causes gut dysbiosis by opening the gut barrier. LPS also causes an increase in blood-brain barrier (BBB) permeability, leading to neuroinflammation (brain and nervous system inflammation). According to *Gut Pathogens*, "A leaky gut allows for the translocation of LPS, molecules found on the outer membrane of Gram-negative bacteria, from the gut into the circulation. LPS, in turn, activates various immune cells, leading to the increased secretion of pro-inflammatory cytokines and low-grade systemic inflammation."[55]

High concentrations of LPS have also been linked to autoimmune disorders, especially in people with inflammatory bowel disease. Elevated levels of LPS indicating leaky gut, as well as dysbiosis, both of which contribute to brain inflammation and neurotransmitter imbalance, have been found in people with autism spectrum disorder.

Blood testing of LPS antibodies, including anti-LPS lgG, lgM, and lgA, can help identify intestinal permeability (paracellular and transcellular) and increased susceptibility to neuroinflammation.

Actin

The protein actin provides barrier structure in the small intestine and controls the assembly and permeability of the tight junctions between epithelial cells. Unhealthy changes in actin lead to increased paracellular permeability.

Anti-actin lgG/lgA includes testing for antibodies against actin, which is associated with the severity of mucosal damage. It is thought that damaged gut tissue results in actin rearrangement and exposure to the gut-associated lymphoid tissue, which triggers an antibody response. This type of immune response has been studied with celiac disease and the resulting intestinal lining damage.

Occludin

Occludin refers to the proteins that link tight junctions between epithelial cells of the small intestine. Elevated blood occludin antibodies, such as IgA, IgM, and IgG, can indicate increased intestinal permeability.

Lactulose/Mannitol Ratio

This test involves orally ingesting the sugars lactulose and mannitol and having your urine collected approximately two to five hours later.[56] Mannitol is a monosaccharide, which is a smaller molecule and is absorbed. Urinary levels of mannitol represent transcellular uptake and absorption. In contrast, lactulose is a disaccharide and larger molecule and should only be slightly absorbed. An elevation of the lactulose to mannitol ratio is a reflection of leaky gut.

Should I Test for Leaky Gut?

It is not essential to be tested for leaky gut. If your health history, signs, and symptoms match up to leaky gut, you can certainly start the holistic protocol in this book and see how you respond. If you are the type of person who likes to see objective data, or you are working with a holistic practitioner who has experience with testing, then you may prefer having a test done. If you do an initial test and then follow my protocols, or those given by your healthcare provider, you can always retest and see the objective improvement. Please be aware that many of the labs that offer leaky gut testing do not accept insurance.

CLINICAL MARKERS FOR DYSBIOSIS

The most direct way to test for dysbiosis is stool analysis. Several companies now offer testing to assess your microbiota balance through DNA analysis as well as the overgrowth of organisms that can become pathogenic. However, microbiome science is still in its infancy, and optimal ranges on testing are still being investigated.[57] There is likely a degree of variation of microbiota, depending on genetics and sex. Nevertheless, like other holistic doctors, I have found microbiome stool testing can help patients by identifying major imbalances in flora, as well as pathogenic microbes.

One other method used by practitioners to test for dysbiosis is called the organic acids urine test. Organic acids are the byproducts of metabolic processes that have occurred in your body. The organic acids pass through more readily than other compounds and can be measured in the urine. There are some markers that can be tested that represent gut dysbiosis, such as intestinal bacteria and yeast. While this test has value, it is more of an indirect test as compared to direct testing of the stool microbiome.

○ ○ ◉ ○ ○

After reading Part I, you now have a good understanding of what leaky gut and dysbiosis involve. In the following chapters I will provide you with all the information I have attained through more than 28 years of practice and treating many thousands of patients, as well as through my research into the most recent science on the subject. I'm excited to share these natural and healing approaches to restoring gut and whole-body health.

PART II

THE HOLISTIC HEALTHY GUT PROTOCOL

Chapter 4

WE ARE THE FOODS
WE EAT AND ABSORB

In Part I, you learned about how your digestive system is critical to your overall health. In particular, the health of your small intestine, where most of your absorption takes place, and the microbiome; it is also the foundation of your immune system activity. Contrary to the phrase "you are what you eat," I expand this concept to "you are the foods you eat and absorb!" The foods that we eat provide the energy and building blocks for our cells and organs. Foods also have an epigenetic effect, meaning they provide information to our DNA (genetics) and affect how the genes express themselves. Healthy foods result in healthier gene expression. In a physical way, foods become a part of us.

Laura, a 22-year-old recent graduate from college, had been experiencing irritable bowel syndrome (IBS) for several years. While she had IBS before college, the diet she consumed and the stress of school had significantly worsened her symptoms. She told me that when she took digestive enzymes and probiotics her symptoms improved. However, if she did not take these supplements for one day, her IBS flared up. I told her that since she did not have the intense stress presently, unlike in college, the key was to improve her diet, because diet changes would work to heal up her leaky gut and dysbiosis in a more permanent way. Laura followed my Modified Mediterranean Diet, and she incorporated one prebiotic or probiotic meal recipe every day. When she followed up with me three months later, she was thrilled to report she had not taken any supplements for the past two months and had no IBS symptoms.

In this chapter and throughout the rest of the book, I will guide you on my time-tested, cutting-edge methods to naturally heal your gut and therefore your body! First, I will take you through the types of foods that heal the gut, such as prebiotics, probiotics, fiber, omegas, fermented foods, and more. We'll also examine those that injure it, such as gluten, sugars, additives, and alcohol, because avoiding these foods can be equally important for gut healing. I'll also explain why following a Mediterranean diet may be the secret to improving your gut health and whole-body health. (My recipes, prepared with a holistic nutritionist, are available in Chapter 9.) Best of all, small changes in diet have a huge impact in a short period of time.

REVITALIZE YOUR INTESTINAL HEALTH

A healthy diet is a foundation for preventing and treating leaky gut. Unfortunately, many people are consuming a diet that promotes a leaky gut. The industrialized Western diet and the Standard American Diet, appropriately abbreviated as SAD, are loaded with processed foods, genetically modified organisms (GMOs), pesticides, and harmful fats and are devoid of healthy flora-feeding fiber as well as nutrients. It is no wonder that so many people are affected by leaky gut. With so many nations adopting the American fast-food diet, we may have a global problem with leaky gut!

Various foods negatively affect the integrity of the small intestine. High-fat diets, alcohol, additives used in the food industry, gliadin (the protein in wheat), food-processing methods using different microbial and fungal strains, and chitosan (a compound from shrimp, lobster, and crabs used as a food preservative) all negatively affect the gut barrier and favor the growth of opportunistic or disease-causing bacteria.[1] Additional research has shown that refined sugars, artificial sweeteners, and a casein-rich (cow's milk protein) diet contribute to leaky gut.[2]

The good news is that the right diet changes can quickly provide the environment for gut healing. I have seen the gut heal in thousands of patients. According to *Gut Pathogens*, "A slight change in the diet can quickly change the gut flora, which in turn can affect the physical and mental well-being of a person."[3] How quick, you ask? Research has shown changes in the microbiota within 48 hours of diet alteration.

GUT-HEALING FOODS

I recommend consuming a diet of foods in their natural state. The more you eat whole foods and restrict processed foods, the better the nutritional composition for gut health. This means eating out less, especially in fast-food restaurants.

In many studies, the Mediterranean diet showed tremendous health benefits for the cardiovascular system, immune system, and brain, as well as reductions in obesity and type 2 diabetes, cancer, inflammation, Alzheimer's disease, depression, onset of Crohn's disease, and mortality. Research has revealed that the Mediterranean diet promotes healthy gut microbiota that has a protective effect against type 2 diabetes.[4] One study reviewed 82 healthy people whose BMI classified them as "overweight" or "obese," and who consumed a low intake of fruit and vegetables and led a sedentary lifestyle. It found that when 43 of the participants switched to a Mediterranean diet for eight weeks, markers of microbiome health improved.[5] The researchers in the study noted that the Mediterranean diet "dynamically modulates the intestinal microbiome composition and that the microbiome variations are proportional to the increase in MD adherence rates." And lastly, researchers conducted a one-year study of more than 600 older people and measured the effects of the Mediterranean diet on the microbiome and other markers.[6] The results of the study found that the Mediterranean diet modulated the gut microbiota in a way that reduced the risk of frailty, improved cognitive function, and reduced inflammation (as measured by inflammation markers like C-reactive protein). I use this diet with many patients because it's a fantastic choice for a lot of people (although everyone is genetically unique and needs to find which diet works best for them).

Prebiotic Foods

You can radically improve your gut health by consuming foods that feed your gut microbiota. Prebiotics refer to nondigestible compounds (mainly nondigestible carbohydrates) metabolized by microorganisms in the gut. Prebiotic foods provide nutrition (energy) for the growth of friendly bacteria in the gut. The health of your gut microbiota depends on the prebiotic foods that you consume. There are a number of different prebiotic foods which include:[7]

- agave
- artichoke
- asparagus
- banana
- barley
- beans
- beet
- chicory
- cocoa-derived flavanols
- honey
- Jerusalem artichoke

- microalgae

- milk (human and cow's milk)

- onion

- peas

- root vegetables

- rye

- seaweeds

- tomato

- whole grain wheat

The Science of Prebiotics

Prebiotics improve intestinal function and health and suppress the growth of disease-causing microbes in the gut by increasing the good bacteria—*Bifidobacterium* and *Lactobacillus*—levels. These friendly floras produce lactic acid, which fights infectious organisms.

When gut microbiota ferments prebiotics, they produce short-chain fatty acids (SCFAs). Examples include lactic acid, butyric acid (butyrate), and propionic acid. There are multiple benefits of these SCFAs in the body, including immune system enhancement and proper colon pH. SCFAs also promote intestinal integrity and reduce inflammation, which protects the intestinal barrier. The short-chain fatty acid known as butyrate has been shown to reduce bacterial movement from the gut to the bloodstream and strengthen intestinal barrier function. SCFAs also reduce the risk for colorectal cancer, irritable bowel syndrome, and Crohn's disease.

The SCFAs produced by prebiotic metabolism in the gut are absorbed through the intestinal cells (enterocytes) and into the bloodstream. Once in the bloodstream, the SCFAs positively affect other organs and systems beyond the digestive system. SCFAs benefits also include:

- development of the nervous system in infants
- improved learning, recall, and memory
- improved immune response
- decreased total and LDL cholesterol, and reduced triglycerides
- lipogenesis (fat breakdown)
- improved calcium absorption
- increased collagen formation
- reduced risk of atopic dermatitis (eczema)[8]

FUNCTIONS OF PREBIOTICS

- Stimulate the growth and reproduction of only useful microflora
- Improve the work of the digestive system
- Maintain an optimal pH in the intestine
- Stimulate peristalsis
- Suppress the reproduction in the intestines of pathogenic bacteria
- Reduce the formation of gases
- Remove excess mucus from the walls of the small intestine

Interesting Inulin

The most consumed prebiotic in its natural form is inulin (also available in supplement form). Food sources include:

- artichoke
- asparagus
- chicory root (as found in coffee substitutes)

- garlic

- green/unripe bananas

- Jerusalem artichoke/sunchoke

- wheat

Inulin helps with weight balance, reduces fasting glucose levels, and decreases liver fat in people with prediabetes. Studies have shown that inulin supplementation improves bowel movement frequency in patients with constipation, reduces gut inflammation, increases beneficial bacteria (*Bifidobacteria*), improves triglyceride and cholesterol levels, and improves the absorption of calcium and magnesium.

Supplementation with inulin should be increased gradually, so the digestive system adjusts to the increased fiber. People with small intestine bacterial overgrowth (SIBO) should avoid supplementation with inulin until their condition is under control.

Gut-Pleasing Polyphenols

Polyphenols refer to compounds found in plants that exert many health benefits. They can be found in many fruits, vegetables, herbs and spices, nuts and seeds, coffee and tea, whole grains, wine, and even chocolate. You may have heard that polyphenols function as powerful antioxidants in the body, preventing cell damage. However, polyphenols have many more health benefits. There are over 8,000 known polyphenols.[9] Studies prove the potential benefits of polyphenols for the prevention and treatment of cardiovascular disease, neurodegenerative disorders, cancer, and obesity. Research has found that polyphenols have a dual benefit to the gut, acting as "duplibiotics," stimulating the growth of friendly flora while selectively reducing harmful bacteria. As a result, polyphenols support a healthy microbiome.

In contrast to the gut-damaging effects of the industrialized Western diet, the Mediterranean diet is rich in polyphenol foods that promote gut healing. It has an abundance of nutrients (glutamine, tryptophan, polyphenols such as quercetin, and curcumin) that promote healthy intestinal permeability.[10]

Fantastic Fiber

Research proves that the average American diet is deficient in fiber: only about 5 percent of the U.S. population consumes enough fiber.[11] According to the Institute of Medicine, fiber needs vary according to age and gender. The recommended total fiber intake (soluble plus insoluble) ranges between 21 to 25 grams for adult females. For adult males, the recommendation is 30 to 38 grams daily. As you will read later in this book, fiber provides the substrate for good bacteria to thrive.

There are two types of fiber—soluble and insoluble—and a healthy diet will include both. Soluble fiber dissolves in water while insoluble does not. Examples of soluble fiber include apples (apple skin), barley, carrots, citrus fruits, oats, beans, and psyllium. When soluble fiber is combined with water, it creates a gel that can improve digestion and bind and reduce cholesterol and blood sugar levels. Insoluble fiber bulks the stool and helps promote regularity. It also binds toxins for excretion from the stool. Examples include wheat, beans, cauliflower, and many vegetables, such as leafy greens. Most plants have a combination of the two types of fiber but vary in their amounts.

A study published in *Nutrients* looked at how dietary fiber affected zonulin levels (a marker of leaky gut) in people with non-alcoholic fatty liver disease.[12] In the study, three portions of vegetables and two portions of fruit were introduced to the patients' diet to include insoluble and soluble foods. Overall, the dietary intake increased from 19 grams daily to 29 grams daily. There was an improvement in blood zonulin levels by nearly 90 percent, suggesting improvement in leaky gut. In addition, there was a significant improvement in liver enzyme levels.

PREBIOTICS TO THE RESCUE

Research has proven that prebiotics can help the following systems of the body:[13]

- *Immune System:* By improving the gut population of friendly and protective microorganisms such as Lactobacilli and Bifidobacteria, the body can better suppress the population of harmful bacteria.

- *Nervous System:* Prebiotics influence the brain through three pathways: the nervous system, endocrine (hormonal), and immune system. Also, prebiotics have been shown to regulate brain growth factors and neurotransmitters (brain chemicals). Additional beneficial effects can be seen with mood, memory, concentration, and learning.

- *Skin:* Prebiotics has been shown to decrease the risk of developing eczema and improve skin hydration.

- *Cardiovascular System:* Prebiotics help the cardiovascular system by reducing inflammation. Studies have also shown improvement in triglyceride and cholesterol levels.

- *Calcium Absorption:* There is scientific evidence that prebiotics increase calcium absorption. Calcium plays a role in many systems of the body, including the bones, muscles, nervous systems, and acts as a critical molecular messenger in our cells.

Safety of Prebiotics

Prebiotic supplements are extremely safe. Higher doses may cause digestive upset in some people, but this can be avoided by gradually increasing the prebiotic amount over several weeks, so the digestive system can adjust to the fiber compounds.

Friendly flora from food and supplements is essential for colonization that prevents the growth of disease-causing bacteria, strengthens the healthy intestine mucus layer, and supports a healthy intestinal barrier structure. An imbalance in the gut flora, known as dysbiosis, results in higher levels of pathogenic bacteria and, thus, higher levels of LPS, damaging intestinal cells and increasing permeability.

Dietary fiber found in grains, fruits, vegetables, and legumes function as prebiotics and are metabolized by gut bacteria into SCFAs, which are important for promoting intestinal integrity and reducing inflammation, protecting the intestinal barrier. The short-chain fatty acid known as butyrate reduces bacterial movement from the gut to the bloodstream and strengthens intestinal barrier function. One of the causes of abnormal SFCS levels is dysbiosis.

Prebiotics and probiotics prevent disease-causing bacteria and fungi from inhabiting the gut and causing permeability. For example, research shows that probiotics prevent *Candida albicans* (fungal organism) from effectively sticking to the gut wall.[14] Also, prebiotics and probiotics work to regulate gut immune function.

Probiotic Foods

The National Institute of Health division known as the National Center for Complementary and Integrative Health defines probiotics as "live microorganisms that are intended to have health benefits when consumed or applied to the body."[15] The International Scientific Association for Probiotics and Prebiotics notes that probiotic health benefits go beyond the digestive tract, including oral (mouth and throat), liver, skin, vaginal, and urinary health.[16]

Examples of probiotic-rich foods include:

- kefir
- kimchi
- kombucha
- kvass
- miso
- natto
- sauerkraut

- soft cheeses
- sour pickles
- tempeh
- yakult
- yogurt

There are several ways that probiotics confer beneficial effects in the gastrointestinal tract. The NIH Office of Dietary Supplements outlines the following gut-healing mechanisms of probiotics:

- They inhibit the growth of pathogenic microorganisms in the gastrointestinal tract.
- They support production of bioactive metabolites (e.g., short-chain fatty acids) and reduction of luminal pH in the colon.
- They are involved in vitamin synthesis.
- They support gut barrier reinforcement.
- They are involved in bile salt metabolism.
- They improve enzymatic activity.
- They support toxin neutralization.[17]

The Science of Probiotics

Probiotics, prebiotics, or a combination of both (known as synbiotics), as well as diets that increase friendly flora such as *Lactobacillus*, all decrease bacterial overgrowth, restore the integrity of the intestinal mucosa, and prevent bacteria (LPS) from being absorbed. Probiotics strengthen the tight epithelial junctions and preserve the mucosal barrier function.[18] They also protect the gut mucosa from toxins, allergens, and disease-causing pathogens.

Probiotics give rise to health-benefiting metabolites known as postbiotics. Postbiotics include bacteriocins, organic acids, butyrate, short-chain fatty acids, and hydrogen peroxide. Some of the postbiotics have been shown to inhibit the growth of disease-causing microbes. Postbiotics are known to be non-toxic and non-pathogenic.

The Journal of Food and Drug Analysis reports several applications of probiotics that may confer many health benefits. These include:

- angiogenic activity (wound healing and repair of damaged tissues)
- anti-pathogenic activity
- anti-obesity activity
- anti-diabetic activity
- anti-allergic activity
- anti-cancer activity
- source of vitamin B
- urogenital healthcare
- positive effect on the brain and central nervous system
- reduction in blood pressure
- cholesterol normalization
- improved lactose metabolism and digestion of food
- boosted immunological response and protection from parasitic infections[19]

Probiotics are measured in what is known as colony-forming units (CFUs). CFU refers to the viable number of cells. Most probiotic supplements contain at least one billion or more CFUs per serving. Depending on the patient and their health situation, I normally use human-studied strains of probiotics in the range of 5 billion to 100 billion CFUs per serving.

Probiotic supplements are extremely safe. The NIH Office of Dietary Supplements states that common probiotic strains "are unlikely to cause harm" and "side effects of probiotics are usually minor and consist of self-limited gastrointestinal symptoms, such as gas."[20] Several studies have looked at the safety of probiotics. A meta-analysis of 17 randomized control trials of patients with irritable bowel syndrome reported overall good safety and tolerance of probiotics.[21] A critical analysis of probiotic supplementation published in *Biomedicine & Pharmacotherapy* deemed probiotics to be safe for healthy people.[22] It noted concern for people with underlying medical conditions, such as those with weakened immune systems and systemic infections. A different paper reviewed 65 randomized controlled trials in regard to probiotics or synbiotics in critically ill adults and children.[23] Of the 18 trials that documented serious adverse events, there were two trials that reported some events. And lastly, a study published in *BMC Gastroenterology* found that probiotic foods and supplements given with the right strain and dose could be effective for the prevention of antibiotic-associated diarrhea.[24] The takeaway message from this research is to have medical guidance for the use of probiotics and synbiotics if you are immune compromised, have serious systemic illness, or are hospitalized.

Postbiotics

Many of you have probably never heard the term *postbiotic*. If you break the word down from its Greek origins, the term *post* means "after" and *bios* means "life." According to *Nutrients*, postbiotic refers to "substances derived after the microorganisms are no longer alive, or, in other words, inanimate, dead or inactivated."[25] In other words, postbiotics are the dead or inactivated parts of friendly flora that can have health benefits. This can include substances such as metabolites produced by probiotics, parts of a microbe's cell wall, proteins or peptides, short-chain fatty acids, enzymes, and other components.

Related to postbiotics is *parabiotics*, also referred to as "inactivated probiotics." These products are "non-viable microbial cells (either intact or ruptured)" that can be given orally or topically for a beneficial effect.[26] Some researchers and authors use postbiotic and parabiotic interchangeably. Other terms for parabiotics include *nonviable probiotics, killed probiotics, ghost probiotics,* and *modified probiotics.* I mention the term *parabiotic* so that you are not confused if you see it on a product label or in an article. For our purposes the term is the same as postbiotic.

One of the ways postbiotics can be made is by fermenting probiotics and then using the metabolites formed. Additional techniques include lab technologies that alter the cell structure of microbes or their physiological function. Researchers have stated that although postbiotics do not contain live microorganisms, they have similar health benefits to those of probiotics.

The Science of Postbiotics

In the book *Precision Medicine for Investigators, Practitioners and Providers*, researchers revealed that there have been approximately 60 randomized controlled trials that have evaluated the safety and efficacy of postbiotics.[27] Studies have been conducted with infants, children, and adults. *Beneficial Microbes* published a meta-analysis involving 40 trials using paraprobiotics (probiotics), comparing them to a placebo, the same living probiotic strain, or only standard therapies.[28] Researchers found similar results to that of the same living probiotic in 86 percent of trials that were focused on prevention of disease and 69 percent of trials focused on treatment of various diseases.

The entire mechanisms of action for postbiotics and parabiotics are not completely known, although they seem to be similar to probiotics. Research demonstrates exciting health benefits for postbiotics, including:

- modulation of the immune system
- prevention of infection
- metabolism of lipids and cholesterol
- anti-tumor activity
- anti-allergy activity
- antioxidant activity
- autophagy (breakdown and destruction of old or damaged cells so there can be renewal with new cells)
- wound healing[29]

In addition, researchers have shown that postbiotics can enhance the intestinal barrier function and mucosal immunity.

Some researchers argue that postbiotics are safer than probiotics, but I would say they are both safe to include in the diet and in supplement form. I recommend you consume prebiotic and probiotic foods most days of the week. I have provided prebiotic and probiotic recipes in the last chapter to make this easier for you. If you have gut problems, then in addition to consuming foods containing prebiotics and probiotics, you can also benefit from daily supplementation of these.

The Omega Factor

The right amount and balance of polyunsaturated fatty acids are essential for preventing and treating leaky gut. Omega-3 fatty acids found in cold water fish (salmon, herring, sardines), nuts and seeds (flaxseed, chia, walnuts), and plant oils (flax and extra virgin olive oil) reduce inflammation. Research in the *International Journal of Molecular Sciences* found that polyunsaturated fatty acids function as precursors to anti-inflammatory compounds to enhance intestinal integrity by regulating tight junction functions.[30]

The other members of polyunsaturated fatty acids are the omega-6 family. Examples include safflower oil, sunflower seeds, walnuts, and pumpkin seeds. However, most people get enough omega-6s from cooking oils in packaged foods and eating out.

It is important to consume enough omega-3 fatty acids in the diet and supplement omega-3s if you do not consume cold water fish on a regular basis. I test patients' blood levels of omega-3 and omega-6, and their relative balance, to see if they have an optimal intake and balanced ratio. I commonly find patients are low in omega-3s.

Supplemental omega-3s include fish oil, flax oil, algae-derived omega-3s, and perilla seed oil. A general amount to supplement is a daily intake of 1000 mg of EPA and DHA combined. These are two of the active omega-3s.

Cool Curcumin

Curcumin is a compound found in the spice turmeric, and research has shown it has a healing effect on the intestinal barrier. Curcumin is taken up by the intestinal epithelial cells and modulates pathways that normally cause leaky gut via inflammation.[31] It also enhances the activity of intestinal alkaline phosphatase and decreases the gut-damaging effects of LPS (discussed in Chapter 1). For this benefit I would use organic turmeric powder at a dose of 1 teaspoon daily in foods or a protein shake.

Fermented Foods

Fermented foods have a long history—their original use was to extend preservation to prevent spoilage. The most common examples in the United States are yogurt and cheese. Other common fermented foods include kefir, kombucha, sauerkraut, tempeh, natto, miso, kimchi, wine, beer, cider, and sourdough bread.

The general process of food fermentation involves microorganisms, such as yeast (e.g., saccharomyces cerevisiae) and bacteria (e.g., *Lactobacillus*), that metabolize foods such as the starch and sugars in plant products to produce organic acids, carbon dioxide, and alcohol in an anerobic condition. The byproducts of alcohol and organic acids increase the acidity of the food and prevent the growth of other microorganisms. There are two main types of fermentation. The first is naturally occurring fermentation, also known as "wild ferments" or "spontaneous ferments." This is the action of microorganisms present in raw food, such as sauerkraut, kimchi, and various fermented soy products. The second type of food fermentation is using starter cultures, also referred to as "culture-dependent ferments," which are added to raw foods, such as in kombucha.

The fermentation process can be applied to most any food that contains plant and animal materials. The popularity of fermented foods is global, and the types depend on the region. In South and East Asia and Southern India, fermented legumes, vegetables, fish, and meat are common. In East Asia, Northern India, Europe, and North America, fermented dairy, meat products, and cereals are more common. In the regions of Africa and South America, inhabitants regularly consume fermented seeds, legumes, milk, and meat products.

The consumption of fermented foods has a modulating or balancing effect on the gut microbiome.[32] Fermented foods themselves contain a large and diverse microbiome. Several studies have been conducted that demonstrate a healthier microbiome diversity in people who consume fermented foods as compared to people who do not.[33] Many but not all of these studies were done with fermented dairy products.

Another benefit of fermented foods is that they increase polyphenol bioavailability. As I stated earlier in this chapter, polyphenols support the growth of healthy flora. In addition, fermented foods increase the production of SCFAs, when fiber is broken down by microbes. The SCFAs also support a healthy gut microbiome and intestinal mucosa. One example of a SCFAs produced by fermentation is acetate. Vinegar is an example of a fermented food that contains high levels of acetate. Various cheeses are also sources of SCFAs.

Researchers have shown that fermented foods are more easily digested, as they partially digest protein by producing enzymes that break down food. Moreover, fermented foods release bioactive peptides, which have health benefits. They also reduce compounds that prevent the absorption of nutrients. And lastly, *The Journal of Nutrition* reported that studies suggest that fermented food consumption supports metabolic and immune-mediated diseases.[34]

I recommend consuming two or more of the fermented food products listed (with the exception of alcohol) on a regular basis. If you are dairy sensitive, there are numerous non-dairy fermented products available on the market. For example, most mornings I consume coconut or macadamia nut yogurt.

FASTING YOUR WAY TO GUT HEALTH

Let's discuss the benefits of fasting to improve gut health. People have fasted for better health and spiritual reasons for thousands of years. In terms of digestive health, fasting allows for the intestinal cells and organs to rest for a period. Animal research has shown that fasting allows the small intestinal villi to remodel (heal). In recent years intermittent fasting, where you abstain from food for 16 to 48 hours, has become popular.

In a 10-day study of 15 healthy men between the ages of 18 and 70 years who followed a medically supervised fast (known as the Buchinger Wilhelmi fasting program) for 10 days, lab testing demonstrated that gut permeability was shown to improve during fasting and remained improved during the refeeding period.[35] In another study, researchers found that obese women following a four-week, very-low-calorie diet (800 calories per day) had markers of gut permeability significantly improved.[36]

Fasting can be a part of your gut-healing protocol. If you are in good health, then intermittent fasting, such as eating in an 8- to 12-hour period each day, or fasting one day a week with water or water/vegetable juice, can be a good choice. If you have diabetes, cancer, heart disease, hypoglycemia, kidney disease, or other serious diseases, then you need to consult with your healthcare provider before undergoing fasting protocols.

PROBLEMATIC FOODS

Now that we've reviewed the foods that heal the gut, it's important to know which foods injure the gut. You want to simultaneously consume foods that help your gut while restricting or avoiding foods that harm your gut. By addressing both components of your diet, you will improve quicker and more fully.

The Gluten Glitch

As mentioned in Chapter 3, gluten is problematic for many people with leaky gut, because it causes changes in zonulin activity and increases intestinal permeability. Gluten is composed of a group of proteins (prolamins and glutelins) and is found in grains like wheat (gliadin and glutenins), rye (secalins and secalinins), and barley (hordeins and hordenins). These proteins are difficult to digest due to their high praline and glutamine content and cause harmful changes in the intestinal barrier, resulting in leaky gut. And as I mentioned earlier, there is emerging evidence that the herbicide glyphosate in our grain supply may be causing an immune system reaction to gluten.

The proteins in gluten resist the digestive protein enzymes (peptidases) produced by the body, making it difficult for them to break down.[37]

A gluten allergy (celiac disease) affects about 1 percent of people worldwide. However, many more people experience non-celiac gluten sensitivity or non-celiac wheat sensitivity. Conventional sources note that an additional 6 percent of the population have one of these sensitivities.[38] However, other nutritional authorities say that the number may be much higher, ranging from 25 percent to 90 percent of the population. I have noticed that many patients feel better and have gut biomarker improvements on a diet that restricts gluten. Many people with a gluten allergy or sensitivity also have challenges with cow's milk products. This is why the Modified Mediterranean Diet at the end of this book is dairy and gluten free.

You should be aware that while a gluten-free diet helps many people with digestive and systemic symptoms and promotes leaky gut healing, there are two downsides. The lack of wheat fiber products makes you susceptible to dysbiosis, in which the level of good bacteria such as *Lactobacillus* and *Bifidobacteria* is too low relative to pro-inflammatory bacteria. Also, the diversity of good bacteria is usually lower in the guts of those on a gluten-free diet. This makes it especially important to include prebiotic and probiotic foods and supplements if you are following a gluten-free diet, especially long-term. The second downside is that whole wheat is a good source of fiber. Fortunately other non-gluten-containing grains can be consumed for fiber such as quinoa, buckwheat, brown rice, non-GMO corn, and others.

Sugars That Feed Gut Pathogens

A remarkably interesting but concerning cascade of events occurs with excess consumption of simple sugars. First, the problem with refined sugars, as found in most pastries, candies, sodas, breads, and pastas, is that they fuel disease-causing microbes in the intestines. These simple sugars also fuel pathogenic bacteria and fungi such as *Candida albicans* and reduce healthy bacteria. Studies with mice have shown that a high-sugar diet (glucose and fructose) increases intestinal permeability.[39]

Second, the overgrowth of these potential pathogen microbes causes toxins (exotoxins) to inflame gut tissue, and malabsorption occurs, leading to undigested proteins being absorbed. And third, these undigested proteins function as antigens, which summon an immune response by the gut-associated lymphoid tissue (GALT).

Fourth, the small intestine villi are destroyed, resulting in losing the enzymes required to digest food. And last, the undigested carbohydrates move further in the intestine and feed pathogenic bacteria, leading to fermentation and leaky gut symptoms.

In order to starve gut pathogens, one must restrict sugars in one's diet.

Artificial Food Ingredients

Research published in the journal *Nutrients* reported that the common food additives may contribute to dysbiosis and inflammation of the gut.[40]

Artificial sweeteners, such as saccharin, sucralose, aspartame, advantame, acesulfame-potassium, and neotame, are known to be 30 to 13,000 times sweeter than sugar (sucrose). Preliminary research shows that these non-natural sweeteners contribute to gut dysbiosis.[41] Therefore, artificial sweeteners should be avoided to ensure optimal gut microbiota health.

Alcohol

If you don't have digestive problems, you should still consume alcohol in moderation, because it increases unhealthy gut bacteria and fungi overgrowth in the gut and creates inflammation. Research shows that alcohol causes the accumulation of endotoxins (toxins formed in the gut) and acetaldehyde in the gut.[42] Acetaldehyde increases gut permeability, allowing endotoxins to be absorbed in the bloodstream and promoting inflammation. Alcohol also imbalances the microbiome.[43] If you have leaky gut or suspect you may have leaky gut, I highly recommend avoiding alcohol altogether until healing has occurred.

Food Sensitivities

As a holistic doctor I have found that food sensitivities, also known as food intolerances, are problematic for some people with gut problems. Please note that I am discussing food sensitivities (intolerances) and not food allergies. A sensitivity can result in unpleasant symptoms that affect the digestive system and other systems of the body, such as a headache, fatigue, muscle aches, foggy brain, or skin rash. An allergy on the other hand is a reaction by the body that can cause very serious or life-threatening symptoms, such as difficulty breathing or hives.

A recent study found a strong association between food sensitivity reactions (IgG) and elevated intestinal markers such as LPS and anti-occludin antibodies.[44] Therefore, identifying and restricting food sensitivities may help in the healing of leaky gut. Blood tests are available through various labs to identify food sensitivities.

You should not experiment with testing known food allergies as they can be life threatening. However, food sensitivities can change and often respond well to nutritional therapies. If you suffer from multiple food sensitivities, then it is probable that you have leaky gut syndrome. Your immune system is hyper-reacting to food particles at the small intestine lining as well as those that enter the bloodstream. If you follow the gut-healing protocols in this book then you will likely find that over time the number and severity of food sensitivities will improve—in many cases dramatically.

You can identify delayed food sensitivities by following an elimination diet, where you stop consuming common foods like gluten, dairy, citrus, corn, soy, and eggs for a period, such as four to six weeks. You can stop all these foods or pick one or two at a time. If you notice improvement by avoiding certain foods, then they are likely problematic. You can also reintroduce the food and see if it is causing problems. Many people find that by healing their leaky gut and dysbiosis (by following the program in this book) their food sensitivities either improve or disappear completely. If your food sensitivities remain after several months, then they may be more genetically caused. In that case restricting them from your diet can promote a healthier gut barrier. In Chapter 9 of this book, I provide you with prebiotic and probiotic recipes as well as a couple of weeks of a Modified Mediterranean Diet to help heal your gut and feed your friendly flora.

○ ○ ◎ ○ ○

Now that you have a better sense of gut-healing foods, you can begin to incorporate them into your diet. You can also eliminate problematic foods and those you have a sensitivity to or have trouble digesting. In the next chapter I'll review all the best supplements for healing leaky gut and dysbiosis. These supplements accelerate gut healing and are valuable in normalizing your gut health.

Chapter 5

SUPER SUPPLEMENTS
FOR LEAKY GUT
AND DYSBIOSIS

Fawn, a 64-year-old woman, had been struggling with gas, bloating, multiple food sensitivities, and fatigue for several years. She was underweight and felt depressed because her diet was so limited. She was wondering if there were other foods she should avoid that were causing problems. My response surprised her—I told her we needed to increase the number of foods that she ate for better diversity of nutrients. However, the first plan of action was to treat her leaky gut and dysbiosis, as that was the underlying cause for her digestive symptoms and overreactive immune system to so many foods. Fawn was both hopeful and nervous about my plan. She was hopeful since I had a plan to help her and what I said made sense, especially in light of the fact that nothing else had helped her. But she was anxious too, since reacting to foods made her feel poorly. After two months of treating her with my protocol, including the use of a gut wellness formula containing glutamine, DGL licorice root, slippery elm, marshmallow root, aloe vera extract, and quercetin, Fawn tried a few new foods without any problem. After the third month she and her husband were delighted to find that she was eating foods she had not consumed in years! In addition, her weight and energy were noticeably improved.

The use of digestive-specific supplements is a powerful way to expedite gut healing, since they augment the body's healing system. These supplements balance the microbiome as well as assist the body in the repair of leaky gut, and they are readily available. I have used the supplements described in this chapter with many thousands of patients throughout my nearly 30 years of practice. Remember, these supplements work best when combined with a healthy diet and lifestyle. My experience is that the correct use of supplements can greatly accelerate the healing process for leaky gut and dysbiosis.

ALOE GETS AN A+

When many people hear the word *aloe,* they think of the cactus-like plant gel used topically to soothe the skin from sunburn. However, aloe has an extensive history for the internal treatment of various conditions, especially conditions of the digestive tract. There are more than 360 species of aloe. The form of aloe most used in North America is aloe barbadensis. Food-grade aloe vera with the laxative components removed (the FDA has banned the use of aloe latex as a laxative) is often prescribed as a supplement by nutrition-oriented doctors.

Aloe vera has antioxidant and anti-inflammatory properties when consumed, which can be important for protecting the gut lining. Also, aloe contains more than 75 compounds, including vitamins A, C, E, and B_{12}; the minerals zinc, copper, and selenium; and enzymes and other compounds. Research published in the *Journal of Complementary and Integrative Medicine* demonstrated that the oral consumption of aloe vera gel extract for 14 days doubled the blood antioxidant capacity of 53 healthy participants.[1]

Participants in the study did not have any allergic reactions or side effects. Aloe contains polysaccharides (sugar chains), which have been shown to inhibit ulcer formation and have a protective effect on colitis.[2] Moreover, aloe vera gel was shown to improve markers of leaky gut in old mice.[3]

Aloe vera can also have the unique effect of reducing the frequency of gastroesophageal reflux (GERD) symptoms. A study published in the *Journal of Traditional Chinese Medicine* reported benefit for people consuming aloe vera syrup (10 ml per day), including reduced heartburn, food regurgitation, dysphagia, flatulence, belching, nausea, and acid regurgitation, with a high degree of safety.[4] In the study, people with GERD were randomized to receive either aloe extract or the GERD drugs ranitidine and omeprazole. The benefits of receiving aloe were comparable to the commonly used GERD medications. Moreover, the study acknowledged that aloe has strong antibacterial effects against *H. pylori*, a bacterium known to infect the stomach and cause gastritis and GERD. In addition, aloe reduces stomach acid secretion, which is helpful for GERD. Unlike common GERD drugs, there is no withdrawal effect when stopping aloe use.

Aloe vera has been shown to have anti-inflammatory effects for colitis and peptic ulcers (ulcers of the first part of the small intestine known as the duodenum). Research in the *Journal of Neurogastroenterology and Motility* revealed that aloe vera was effective in three randomized controlled trials in relieving irritable bowel syndrome as compared to placebo.[5] There were no serious adverse events in these trials.

I have seen good results with standardized food-grade aloe powders and liquids for many years. I mainly use concentrated aloe in combination with licorice (DGL) and glutamine, blended in a powder form so that the ingredients come into contact with the esophagus, stomach, small intestine, and colon. Since formulas vary, follow the instructions on the label for dosage.

LOVING LICORICE

Licorice is a widespread ingredient in herbal therapies used by practitioners worldwide. It has been particularly revered in Ayurvedic and TCM, as well as in European herbal medicine practices. The traditional uses of licorice are many, including the treatment of digestive ailments such as ulcers and abdominal pain. There are different species of licorice that are used medicinally.

The form I have used with patients for several decades, and one common in European and North American herbalism, is *Glycyrrhiza glabra*. Licorice has anti-inflammatory, antimicrobial (including antiprotozoal), antioxidant, liver-protective, and nervous system–balancing activities, and it's effective in treating dyspepsia.[6]

Licorice stimulates mucin secretion by the stomach and intestines.[7] Remember, mucin is a protective barrier in the small intestine. It is a common mucus protein secreted by specialized cells (goblet cells) in the small and large intestine. This mucus layer acts as a physical defense against toxins and bacteria, preventing them from contacting the intestinal barrier.

The form of licorice that is mainly used in holistic medicine is deglycyrrhizinated licorice, known as DGL. This supplemental form of licorice removes the component that may elevate blood pressure in some individuals, especially at higher doses.

DGL increases blood flow to the damaged mucosa of the gut and is effective for treating small intestine (duodenal) ulcers.[8] DGL also contains flavonoids, which have anti-inflammatory effects and have shown to protect against ulcers in animal studies. Moreover, DGL increases intestinal life span, another protective effect.

Published research has shown that DGL was similar or more effective than common anti-ulcer drugs for the treatment of ulcers. In addition, animal studies have shown that licorice protects against ulcers induced by aspirin.[9] Licorice (*Glycyrrhiza glabra*) also provides anti-inflammatory and antioxidant effects on the mucosa lining of the digestive tract, which helps intestinal disorders.[10]

DGL protects against damage to the small intestine barrier and tight junction proteins and reduces inflammatory markers known to cause gut damage.[11] This is the effect we would want in preventing and treating leaky gut.

DGL is available as chewable tablets (1 to 2 tablets) and powder form (use as directed on the label). It is best to take it before meals. Regular licorice root can also be used, especially in formulas, although high doses should be avoided unless under the guidance of a holistic practitioner.

GLUTAMINE—GUT FUEL FOR YOUR INTESTINES

Glutamine is the most abundant free amino acid in the body. Your body can make glutamine, but you may need to acquire it through food. If your diet is deficient or you have malabsorption conditions, taking supplements can be beneficial. The intestines use about one-third of the total glutamine in the body, and they need glutamine more than any other organ. Glutamine is a fuel source for intestinal cells, and it decreases small intestine cell damage, and supports gut function and the integrity of the gut mucosa.[12]

The *International Journal of Molecular Sciences* explained the roles of glutamine for intestinal health as follows: This amino acid has been shown to prevent premature cell death (apoptosis) of the intestinal cells. The intestinal cells turn over every three to four days, a type of regenerative effect. Premature death of intestinal cells occurs in conditions like ulcerative colitis or bacterial infections. Glutamine prevents premature apoptosis by functioning as a precursor to the antioxidant glutathione, regulating the enzymes and proteins involved in apoptosis, controlling inflammation, and decreasing cellular stress, as well as regulating the breakdown and replacement of intestinal cells (autophagy).[13]

If glutamine stores are deficient, the intestinal lining is vulnerable to damage. Glutamine plays a vital role in gut health. It is a preferred substance for intestinal cell replication. Like most other cells in the body, the intestinal cells replace old cells with new cells. *Frontiers in Nutrition* reported that glutamine promotes healthy small intestine cell proliferation, regulates tight junction proteins, reduces inflammatory pathways, and promotes healthy microbiota by regulating the gut bacteria utilization of amino acids.[14] It also revealed that glutamine supplementation was helpful in lessening the symptoms of IBS when combined with a low-FODMAP diet.

Glutamine is a nutrient-specific amino acid for the support of gut cell turnover. According to *Current Opinion in Clinical Nutrition & Metabolic Care*, "Glutamine is a major nutrient to maintain intestinal function in animals and humans."[15] It also reported that the depletion of glutamine damages the small intestine villi, where much of the absorption occurs. Glutamine favors the health of tight junction proteins by increasing protein synthesis, decreasing oxidative stress and inflammation, and possibly modifying gut bacteria. And last, glutamine can activate enzymes that support intestinal stem cells and growth factors that repair intestinal cells.

Glutamine is available in supplement form in capsules, tablets, and powders. I generally recommend powder form to ensure contact with the amino acid and the gut mucosa. I typically have patients take 2000 to 5000 mg a day of glutamine powder for leaky gut treatment. Higher doses can be used as well.

QUERCETIN QUASHES INFLAMMATION

Quercetin is a compound found in edible plants that have potent anti-inflammatory and antioxidant properties. Common quercetin-containing foods in the Western diet include vegetables (onions, asparagus, green peppers, tomatoes, red leaf lettuce), tea, red wine, and fruits (apples, berries, grapes).

Quercetin can benefit gut-healing because it reduces the release of histamines and other pro-inflammatory compounds (cytokines, leukotrienes, and others). Chronic inflammation, including in the gut, leads to tissue breakdown and damage. Quercetin, through its activity as an antioxidant and stabilizer of mast cell histamine release, may improve gut health.

Mast cells are immune cells found throughout the body but within the highest concentration in the digestive tract. According to *Immunobiology*, "Mucosal mast cells are primary regulators of the physical integrity and function of the intestinal epithelial barrier."[16] Mast cells are activated during allergic and inflammatory reactions, and they release inflammatory chemicals. The release of chemicals such as histamine can also lead to an inflammatory response in the gut, and long-term activation of histamine can lead to increased permeability. Quercetin has been shown to stabilize mast cells and attenuate histamine release. It suppresses inflammatory chemicals (cytokines), improves antibody production in the gut, and enhances the growth of friendly flora.[17]

Nutrients revealed that "quercetin enhances intestinal barrier function and modulates microbiota composition."[18] It explained that quercetin promotes the assembly of tight junctions, remodels the tight junctions, and enhances barrier integrity. It also reported that quercetin is fermented by gut microbiota in the intestine to produce short-chain fatty acids. These mechanisms are helpful for healing leaky gut.

A study published in *The Journal of Nutrition* showed that quercetin enhanced the barrier function of human intestinal cells.[19] The beneficial effect of quercetin in this study was on its ability to promote the assembly of the proteins involved in the tight junctions of intestinal cells.

Quercetin is very safe and well tolerated. For the long-term treatment of leaky gut, I recommend 50 to 100 mg of the phytosome form.

SLIPPERY ELM SOOTHER

The bark of slippery elm (*Ulmus fulva*) has a long history of medicinal use in North America. Slippery elm contains mucilage, which when combined with water results in a slick gel that coats and soothes the throat and intestines.[20] This plant also improves gastrointestinal mucus that may protect against ulcers.

Slippery elm is a time-tested natural remedy. It contains anti-oxidants, which benefit inflammatory bowel conditions.[21] One study reported that slippery elm exhibits antioxidant properties that may have anti-inflammatory effects that should be considered for the treatment of inflammatory bowel disease.[22]

Slippery elm can be taken in the forms of capsules, teas, lozenges, and powders. I most often use it in the powder form, but any of these forms can be effective.

MARVELOUS MARSHMALLOW ROOT

Another time-tested plant remedy for the digestive tract is marshmallow root (*Althaea officinalis*). Dr. Tilgner, author of *Herbal Medicine*, reported that marshmallow root "is used for soothing mucous membrane irritation in the gastrointestinal tract. . . ."[23] She noted that marshmallow root can act as an antispasmodic and anti-inflammatory. Like slippery elm, it contains mucilage, which is soothing to the gut mucosa. According to the *Journal of Ethnopharmacology*, the polysaccharides of marshmallow root have healing effects on the activity of epithelial cells, and this effect is in accordance with its traditional use.[24] Antioxidants found that marshmallow root reduced mucosal irritation and ulceration in an animal study.[25]

Marshmallow root is very safe and can be taken in the forms of capsules, teas, lozenges, and powders. I most often use it in the powder form, but any of these forms can be effective.

DIGEST WITH DIGESTIVE ENZYMES

The technology to supplement digestive enzymes with meals has been around for several decades. Digestive enzyme supplements are designed to mimic and assist with the body's production of digestive enzymes, especially those of the pancreas. In terms of leaky gut, the better we break down and digest our food, the less irritation that is caused in the small intestine lining. Nutrients can be absorbed better and the body becomes healthier, including the small intestine. In terms of research, *Nutrients* reported that leaky gut contributes to undigested food fragments, which may act as pro-inflammatory agents that cause immune system dysfunction as they enter the blood circulation of the body.[26] Therefore, you can see the importance of not only eating healthy but also having proper digestion of food.

There are different types of digestive enzymes. Prescription digestive enzymes are known as exogenous pancreatic enzymes. These types of enzymes are normally prescribed by doctors in a limited number of conditions, such as exocrine pancreatic insufficiency (a condition characterized by fat in the stool, weight loss, pancreatic inflammation, and elevated blood pancreatic enzymes). These prescription enzymes are normally derived from pork or beef sources. There are also over-the-counter supplements available that contain pancreatic enzymes. There can be problems with the survivability of pancreatic enzymes in low-pH stomach acid. However, enteric-coated tablets (i.e., those with a coating that protects against stomach acid and allows substances to stay intact until they reach the small intestine) have been shown to work well.

A second category of enzymes are plant enzymes, which include bromelain taken from pineapple and papain from papaya. These enzymes aid in the digestion of protein.

Many doctors like myself use microbial-derived enzymes. These enzymes are generally produced from the fermentation of fungus. For example, fungi such as *Aspergillus oryzae* and *Aspergillus niger* are grown on wheat or rice bran and also given other substances that encourage enzyme activity. Once this occurs, the enzymes go through laboratory purification and then are dried, concentrated, and standardized for their activity (potency). These types of enzymes can be used in formulas to not only break down fats, carbohydrates, and proteins but also for specialty uses such as breaking down gluten (people with celiac disease still need to avoid gluten), sugar, plant fiber, lactose, and other compounds.

A study published in *Clinical Psychopharmacology and Neuroscience* revealed the benefit of supplemental enzymes.[27] The double-blind, randomized clinical trial involved 101 children with autism spectrum disorder who were given either digestive enzymes or a placebo. Researchers found that the group receiving the supplemental enzyme therapy for three months had significant improvement in several categories of testing, including emotional response, general impression autistic score, general behavior, and digestive symptoms.

Research has shown that the stool level of enzymes, known as fecal elastase, are low in people with irritable bowel syndrome–diarrhea type (IBS-D). According to the *Journal of Digestive Diseases*, the use of digestive enzyme supplementation was effective for post-meal diarrhea associated with IBS-D.[28] In addition, other studies have shown digestive enzymes improve other symptoms, including abdominal distention, belching, diarrhea, abdominal pain, epigastric burning, flatulence, bloating, belching, a feeling of fullness, and loss of appetite.

Enzymes are quite safe to use. High protein–activity enzymes should be used with caution for those with active ulcers. The typical recommendation is one to two capsules or tablets taken with regular meals to aid digestion.

BITTERS ARE BEAUTIFUL

Bitters in herbal medicine refer to herbs that have a bitter taste and are often used to improve digestion. There is a long history of their use for medicinal effects in Traditional Chinese Medicine as well as European and North American naturopathic herbal therapy. In the early 20th century the medical profession recognized that bitters improved digestion.[29] Some bitter herbs are toxic, so only consume those that have proven medicinal uses.

Common bitter herbs you may be aware of include dandelion root, wormwood, and gentian root. Liquid bitters formulas are easy to find and often contain a blend of bitter herbs; you may be able to find some bitters in capsule form as well. Coffee and some alcohol beverages are bitter and are known to stimulate digestive action too.

There are a few ways that bitter herbs stimulate digestion.[30] One type of physiological reaction is the stimulation of bitter receptors in the mouth and throat that then causes a nervous system response to increase saliva production and vagus nerve stimulation of the digestive organs. The authoritative German Commission E supports this mechanism of action. Another reaction can involve the bitters stimulating receptors of the mouth and throat and digestive organs directly upon contact. And last, bitters improve blood circulation in the abdominal organs, which supports digestion through the production of digestive juices, movement of food, absorption of nutrients, and removal of metabolic wastes. In Chapter 3 I discussed one of the root causes of leaky gut, which was decreased blood and nerve flow to the gut. It should be noted that the German Commission E supports the first physiological model I described.

Interestingly, research reveals that there are indeed bitter receptors throughout the GI tract,[31] not only in the mouth but also throughout the digestive tract on enteroendocrine cells. These receptors are also in the stomach, intestine, and pancreas. When activated, the sensors receive bitter signals and then release hormones involved in the digestion and absorption of food. There are more than 25 different types of taste receptors that detect bitterness in the human body.

While there may be advantages to tasting bitters in liquid form, the research demonstrates that the capsule form of bitters works as well. For example, *Nutrients* found that the capsule form of hops extract (a bitter) stimulates the release of cholecystokinin (CCK).[32] CCK is a digestive hormone produced by small intestine cells that is released into the blood when we eat. CCK binds to the receptors of digestive organs, such as the gallbladder, pancreas, and stomach, to stimulate activity of digestion and absorption.

One of the most common bitter herbs used in supplement form in holistic medicine is gentian root (*Gentian lutea*). Different types of gentian species are used medicinally throughout the world. A German study reported the effect of gentian root in people with various indigestion symptoms, such as heartburn, vomiting, stomachaches, nausea, loss of appetite, constipation, and flatulence.[33] The participants were given 120 mg of gentian root in capsule form at a frequency of 2 to 3 times daily for 15 consecutive days. Thirty-one percent of the participants reported excellent results, 55 percent reported good results, 9 percent reported a moderate benefit, and only 5 percent reported an inadequate response. A commonly used capsule of gentian root and skullcap (*Scutellaria lateriflora*) has been used by naturopathic doctors for many decades as a tonic for a variety of digestive and systemic illnesses.

Bitters are often taken for several weeks or months for people with chronic digestive problems. Bitters seem to "retrain" the digestive system to work more efficiently. For people under chronic stress, bitters can help aid digestion until the stress is under control.

Bitters are generally safe but should not be used in people who have active ulcers or gastritis (although some animal studies found it to be helpful for these conditions). It is best to take bitters before or with meals. Bitters can be used in liquid and capsule form.

PREBIOTICS AND PROBIOTICS

Prebiotics and probiotics (as foods and supplements) are critically important in recovering from leaky gut and dysbiosis. In the previous chapter, I provided a comprehensive review of the benefits of prebiotics, probiotics, and postbiotics, so in this chapter I will focus on the proper use of prebiotic and probiotic supplements. The number of products available in this category is vast.

I always recommend that patients focus on products that have published human studies on the ingredients they are using. Some products have studies on the exact product, while other products contain human-studied components. I see a lot of probiotics on the market that have either no human studies or contain ingredients with human studies but at doses lower than what the published studies used.

Fortunately, there are many good prebiotic and probiotic supplements available on the market. The use of these products is very important for people who are having trouble making adequate diet changes so that prebiotics and probiotics are part of their regular diet. People with leaky gut and dysbiosis will often recover faster when quality products are used in addition to diet changes that incorporate prebiotics and probiotics. Do your research before purchasing prebiotics and probiotics—your holistic healthcare provider can steer you in the right direction for quality products.

COLLAGEN PROTEIN FOR GUT HEALTH

There are more than 25 types of collagens in the human body. Most collagen is made of types 1, 2, and 3, with type 1 being the most common. Type 1 is the form found in the digestive tract. Signs and symptoms of collagen deficiency may include skin, joint, hair, and nail problems, as well as leaky gut. This is why collagen has become a popular supplement to support joint, hair, skin, nail, and digestive health. Collagen is the most abundant protein in the body, accounting for approximately 30 percent of the body's protein.[34] It is the primary building block of the body's skin, muscles, bones, tendons, ligaments, and connective tissues. These biological facts demonstrate that collagen plays an essential role in the structure and function of the human body.

Foods containing the amino acids that may promote collagen formation include fish, poultry, meat, eggs, dairy, legumes, and soy.[35] Foods that provide vitamin C, zinc, and manganese in plants are also important for collagen formation. *Nutrients* cites research that collagen consumption for the average American diet is about 3 grams per day, unless you consume a high amount of sausage and frankfurters, which then increases it to an average of 23 grams per day.[36] This demonstrates the wide array of collagen protein consumption according to dietary habits.

Animal studies have shown that collagen peptides improve intestinal mucosa health and decrease intestinal and whole-body inflammation through a protective effect on the intestinal epithelial barrier function (IEBF).[37] Researchers have also noted that collagen peptides can repair intestinal mucosa dysfunction, including the repair of tight junctions. One of the known reasons why collagen peptides reduce intestinal inflammation and improve IEBG regulation is partly due to the amino acid composition of glycine, arginine, and leucine. Glycine improves the intestinal mucosal barrier, inhibits oxidative stress and inflammation responses, and improves tight junctions. Proline also improves the tight junction proteins, and leucine improves the gut immune response.

Research shows that collagen peptides as found in collagen protein powders are generally safe to use. People with kidney disease should check with their doctor first before using any protein supplements. Use collagen products that have human studies. Typical doses are 5 to 15 grams daily. Use as directed on the container.

ADDITIONAL NUTRIENTS

There are many nutrients that the body uses to control inflammation and maintain cellular health. The *American Journal of Physiology: Gastrointestinal and Liver Physiology* cited research on human and animal studies with regard to gut barrier health and the nutrients A, D, and zinc.[38] It explained that fat-soluble vitamins A and D affect the mucosal wall by playing a role in the integrity of the epithelial layer, the immune systems within the small intestine mucosa (innate and adaptive), and the gut microbiota. Moreover, the nutrients A, D, and zinc play an important role in the health of the tight junction proteins, which regulate small intestine permeability. And lastly, the use of omega-3 supplements is worthy of consideration as a nutrient to support gut health. Increasing food intake of these nutrients and the use of supplements can help accelerate gut healing.

Vitamin A

Vitamin A is found in animal products in a ready-to-use form (retinol) and in fruits and vegetables in the form of carotenoids that can be converted to vitamin A. This fat-soluble vitamin is involved in normal cell division. People with inflammatory bowel disease and celiac disease or other malabsorption conditions are more likely to be deficient in vitamin A.[39]

Vitamin A plays a role in the immune system of the gut mucosal barrier and influences the production of antibacterial proteins. One study in the *Journal of Infectious Diseases* revealed that children deficient in vitamin A found that supplementation improved leaky gut biomarkers.[40]

The recommended amount of supplemental vitamin A is approximately 2500 IU (750 µg). I generally recommend it as part of a high-quality multivitamin.

Vitamin D

Vitamin D is actually a prohormone—a substance that is converted into a hormone, a chemical messenger. When the skin is exposed to ultraviolet B radiation, it forms vitamin D that is then transported to the liver and kidneys to be activated. Vitamin D acts through the vitamin D receptors in the nucleus of the cell and affects the activity of genes. While many people are familiar with vitamin D for its role in the absorption of calcium in the intestines, it plays a much larger role in the body. Vitamin D is involved in cell division and is a potent modulator of the immune system, as well as other roles.

Vitamin D can become deficient in people who are not exposed to sunlight, people with inflammatory bowel diseases and malabsorption issues, those who are obese, those taking certain medications such as proton pump inhibitors for acid reflux or medicine for seizures, and people with magnesium deficiency. There are not many food sources of vitamin D, but it can be found in fish, such as mackerel, salmon, and sardines, mushrooms exposed to sunlight, and fortified foods with vitamin D.

Research in *Autoimmunity Reviews* revealed that vitamin D plays a role in "maintaining the integrity of the intestinal barrier."[41] It reported that vitamin D influences the gut integrity, immune modulation in the gut, as well as composition of the microbiome. It also suggested that there is "strong evidence" that vitamin D signaling to the intestinal epithelial cells is of "great importance" for controlling inflammation in the gut and maintaining intestinal wall health. A three-month study published in the *United European Gastroenterology Journal* found that supplementation of vitamin D (2000 IU daily) for people with stable Crohn's disease resulted improvement in markers of leaky gut.[42]

Many people have a vitamin D deficiency or suboptimal levels of vitamin D. The NIH Office of Dietary Supplements defines vitamin D deficiency as a 25 (OH)D level less than 30 nanomoles/liter and insufficiency or suboptimal levels at 30 to 50 nanomoles/liter.[43] As a reference point, many labs have a vitamin D (25 OH) reference range of 30 to 100 nanomoles/liter. Blood testing can identify vitamin D deficiency. I generally recommend that patients with low levels supplement with 2000 IU (50 mcg) to 5000 IU (125 mcg) of vitamin D_3 daily with food (since it is fat soluble). Most of my patients supplement 5000 IU of vitamin D_3 daily with meals and take it combined with K_2. However, your blood levels will dictate the precise dose.

Zinc

The mineral zinc plays many important roles in the body, including immunity and intestinal ion transport. However, its most important role is its participation in regulating over 50 different enzymes required for cellular chemical reactions.

Zinc deficiency may occur from malabsorption, as seen with inflammatory bowel disease, alcoholism, use of proton pump inhibitors for acid reflux, and for those consuming a vegetarian diet. Food sources include shellfish, red meat, nuts, eggs, and legumes. The recommended daily allowance for males is 11 mg per day and 8 mg for females.[44]

Zinc deficiency leads to a compromised digestive epithelial barrier function.[45] When zinc is deficient, there can be leakiness of the tight junction seals in the epithelial layers of the small intestine.

I typically recommend 15 mg to 25 mg daily of zinc supplementation as part of a multivitamin or by itself when treating leaky gut syndrome.

Omega-3 Fatty Acids

Omega-3 fatty acids are part of the polyunsaturated fatty acids that the body requires through diet since the body cannot make them. The direct sources of omega-3 fats in fish include eicosapentaenoic acid (EPA) and docosahexaenoic acid (DHA). Another type of omega-3 polyunsaturated fatty acids includes alpha-linolenic acid (ALA). ALA is found in nuts, seeds, green leafy vegetables, and beans and can be converted into the more active EPA and DHA.

The *International Journal of Molecular Sciences* reported that omega-3 fatty acids "exert significant effects on the intestinal environment" and have a modulating effect on the gut microbiota.[46] Omega-3s are known to reduce inflammation in various areas of the body, including the digestive tract. Research has shown that omega-3 fatty acids act as a type of prebiotic for healthy gut microbiota.[47]

People with Crohn's disease who take fish oil have reduced disease activity and inflammation. While there have been more animal studies than human studies on the effects of omega-3s on gut health, given the inflammation-reducing effects of omega-3s, people with leaky gut should increase their intake to create an environment conducive to gut healing.

Direct omega-3 supplementation is achieved mainly through fish oil supplements. Contrary to what some medical authorities proclaim, highly purified fish oil is readily available from health food stores and health practitioners. Independent analysis of the purity and potency is made available by many companies. Vegetarian sources of EPA and DHA are also available from omega-3 oils derived from algae, flaxseed, or perilla. I generally recommend 1000 mg of EPA and DHA combined as a daily dose. If you have a sensitive digestive system, then enteric-coated fish oil is available. If you are on anticoagulant therapy, consult with your doctor before supplementing omega-3s.

○ ○ ◎ ○ ○

You can see there are several supplements you can take to help with healing a leaky gut and dysbiosis. One thing to be aware of is that infections in the gut may require special treatment with certain supplements or, in more severe cases, medications. This is something you would need to have tested and treated by a healthcare provider. That being said, I have found most of my patients with leaky gut respond very well to supplementation. On average people take these supplements for three to six months, depending on the severity of their symptoms and how well they change their diet and lifestyle. Some people remain on a lower dose of some of these supplements for ongoing digestive problems, usually due to chronic illness, being unable to correct their diet and lifestyle, or not addressing root causes such as underlying infections (*Candida*, parasites, SIBO, etc.).

I have had great results with formulas containing powders of aloe, DGL, glutamine, quercetin, marshmallow root, and slippery elm. This combination of ingredients targets different mechanisms of healing leaky gut. The soothing, anti-inflammatory, and mucus-regenerative effect of these herbs can provide quick relief for people suffering from acid reflux, abdominal cramping, abdominal spasming, and bouts of diarrhea or constipation. You could certainly take each of these products individually, especially the aloe, DGL, and glutamine to start.

I also advise taking a supplement to aid in the breakdown and digesting of foods. The simplest approach is to take a comprehensive digestive enzyme with all regular meals. However, another great option is bitter herbal formulas before or with meals as I described earlier in this chapter.

Also important is the use of a good probiotic. Choose a probiotic that has been validated by published human studies. Normally probiotics are not taken during meals. If you are having trouble getting enough prebiotics from your diet (there are examples in Chapter 9), then a prebiotic supplement can be helpful.

Last, take a high-quality multivitamin and mineral formula, or a functional food such as a protein shake with the nutrients added to the formula. This provides a broad base of nutrients for gut and immune health.

If you are overwhelmed with taking supplements, start slowly with one or two products and see how you respond. You are on the right track if your digestion and overall health is improving. If you find your improvement is slow, you need to target your gut health with other supplements I have discussed here. The longer you have had leaky gut and dysbiosis, the longer it will take to feel better. However, most of my patients notice an obvious improvement with my protocol within two to four weeks. If you are not improving, you may need additional testing, such as stool testing, to see if there are other reasons for your gut problems.

Chapter 6

THE BEST LIFESTYLE FOR A HEALTHY GUT

Shelly, a 20-year-old college student, came to my clinic for problems with abdominal bloating and cramping. As I talked to her more about when her digestive symptoms began, I found out that they only occurred during the school semesters. During the breaks at home she would not have many symptoms, even when she did not eat well. One of the keys for healing her digestive problems was regular exercise as well as receiving treatment with neurofeedback, which helped her to respond to stress more effectively.

One thing you can be certain of when it comes to gut health is that it is interconnected with the rest of the body. This includes communication between the brain and the gut. As you are aware, the ill effects of stress can contribute greatly to digestive problems, including leaky gut and dysbiosis. This is why a healthy lifestyle that goes beyond diet, supplements, and other therapies mentioned in this book is so important for quick and permanent gut healing.

Researchers have declared stress the "Health Epidemic of the 21st Century."[1] Certainly, many people in healthcare who work with patients would agree with this notion. People from all walks of life feel that their stress level is affecting their health and quality of life in a detrimental way. The WHO defines stress as change that causes strain physically, emotionally, or psychologically. The workplace is a common source of stress. And, certainly, the COVID-19 pandemic was a major source of stress physically, mentally, and emotionally. Unfortunately, the pandemic also increased workplace stress for many people.

Everyone handles stress differently. Often it is not so much the stress itself that is the problem, but more so how we perceive or cope with the stress. This is why different approaches work better or worse depending on our susceptibility and personality. How we respond to stress has major health implications. We all have to deal with stress, and the body has mechanisms designed to adapt and perform under stress. However, if stress is too intense and/or becomes chronic, it can result in an unhealthy biological response. As a result, we become susceptible to various health problems.

HOW MUCH STRESS CAN YOU HANDLE?

Our bodies are designed to quickly adapt to stress. They contain sensors (receptors) all over, including in the brain, to monitor our external and internal environments. When they detect imbalances or threats, they assess and respond. However, there is a limit to the amount of stress we can handle, and it varies depending on the individual.

An article in *Psychological Review* discussed the term *allostasis*, which is used to describe the body's response to stress and can be defined as the process whereby one adapts to change.[2] The other related term often used in the study of the body's response to stress is *allostatic load*. *Psychotherapy and Psychosomatics* defines allostatic load as the cost of being exposed to stress and the adjustments we need to make in response to stress.[3] The key point here is that when the external stressors exceed our ability to cope, allostatic overload occurs. Reasons for overload include exposure to frequent stressors, inability to adapt to the stress, and inability to stop the stress response after the stressor is gone.

Here's a real-life example: A 36-year-old woman named Zola came to my office for integrative cancer support. She'd recently had a lumpectomy for breast cancer and was about to receive chemotherapy followed by radiation. In reviewing her history, I found she had a clean diet, exercised five times a week, did not drink excessively, and never smoked. She also had no strong genetic predisposition to cancer based on her family history and gene testing. She mentioned that during the three years leading up to her diagnosis her stress level was extremely high. She was having concerning problems in her marriage and was close to a divorce. As I revealed in my book *Outside the Box Cancer Therapies*, stress can make your body more susceptible to cancer.[4]

THE STRESS RESPONSE IN YOUR BODY

Perhaps you are one of the many readers suffering from health problems such as leaky gut, and you know that stress has been preventing your health from being restored. Before I get into some of the effective tools you can use for managing stress, I want to review the important role that your brain and adrenal glands play in communicating—to make it possible for our bodies to deal with stress.

The brain has a critical communication system with the adrenal glands that messages almost instantaneously. The adrenal glands are sometimes referred to as the stress glands. Located on top of both kidneys, these specialized endocrine glands produce stress neurohormones (which have neurotransmitter and hormonal messaging actions) such as epinephrine (adrenaline) and norepinephrine (noradrenaline). Additional stress hormones that can have powerful effects on the body include cortisol, DHEA, and others.

The brain communicates with the adrenal glands via hormonal messengers as well as nerve pathways. You likely have heard of the fight-or-flight response. One part of the nervous system is the *sympathetic* system. When parts of the brain such as the hypothalamus receive messages of concern, the sympathetic nervous system sends messaging via the autonomic nerves to the adrenal glands. The short-term response of epinephrine and norepinephrine through nervous system messaging increases heart rate and blood pressure, stimulates the liver to break down glycogen to glucose and release it into the blood for energy supply, dilates bronchioles, reduces digestion and urination, and increases metabolic rate. These actions help us adapt to all different types of stresses.

As the acute stress decreases, the hypothalamus releases messaging through the *parasympathetic* system to calm the response. However, long-term stress keeps the sympathetic nervous system overactivated through messaging with hormones. The hypothalamus releases corticotropin-releasing hormone (CRH), which sends messaging to the pituitary gland (below the hypothalamus and still in the brain), which then releases adrenocorticotropic hormone (ACTH) through the bloodstream to the adrenal glands, resulting in cortisol release. Keep in mind this is a simplified version since additional stress hormones are also being released and activating or deactivating the stress response.

Although there are similarities in the body's response to short-term stress and long-term stress, there is a different cascade of hormones released with long-term stress that makes the body more prone to breakdown. For example, high levels of cortisol over prolonged periods of time lead to a breakdown of the major organ systems of the body, including the brain, digestive tract, cardiovascular system, immune system, and so on. More specific to the digestive system, stress negatively affects absorption, intestinal permeability, mucus and stomach acid secretion, gut motility, appetite, gut bacteria imbalance, and GI inflammation.[5]

Adrenal Dysfunction

You may recognize the term *adrenal fatigue*. This term has been used to indicate weakened or burned-out adrenal glands that cause fatigue and other symptoms. The conventional medical establishment is not supportive of this term. Conventional medicine recognizes rare medical conditions where there is a major deficiency of adrenal hormones, known as primary adrenal insufficiency or Addison's disease. In addition, they recognize excessive cortisol production, known as Cushing's syndrome. The reality is most people experience adrenal hormone imbalance somewhere between low-normal to high-normal. A term that integrative doctors have been using recently, and one I support, is *adrenal dysfunction*. However, as I mentioned earlier, the adrenal glands do not work in isolation. So, the term *adrenal dysfunction* really means imbalanced adrenal hormones as a result of a communication imbalance from the hypothalamus and pituitary glands, also known as the hypothalamic-pituitary-adrenal axis (HPA axis). The term *HPA axis dysfunction* is found in the medical literature. Therefore, the term *adrenal dysfunction* (easier to refer to) is the same as HPA Axis Dysfunction.

One of the best ways to test for adrenal dysfunction is salivary stress hormone testing. This testing involves collecting multiple saliva samples over the course of a day. Saliva testing makes it practical to measure your stress hormone levels multiple times in a day or over several days to see if the hormone levels match a typical pattern. This type of testing is routine in stress studies conducted at major research institutions. Saliva testing is also more convenient and accurate since some people experience stress during a blood draw, which can affect blood cortisol levels. Saliva testing can identify people with irregular cortisol patterns that may be too low, too high, or a mixture. It should be noted that in recent years dried urine testing is being used as well in testing cortisol and other hormone levels. Many tests measure morning DHEA levels in addition to cortisol, which is another adrenal hormone that the body uses to combat the effects of stress and works in tandem with cortisol.

For many people, adrenal dysfunction can be identified by its signs and symptoms. Classic symptoms include fatigue, inability to cope with mental or physical stress, and poor exercise recovery.

Moreover, adrenal dysfunction can be associated with other signs and symptoms, including digestive problems.

Balancing Your Adrenals

Holistic approaches to balancing your HPA axis are by far the best way to optimize adrenal hormones. You will find many people with adrenal dysfunction taking antidepressants, anti-anxiety medications, and recreational drugs to try to cope with their brain and body's poor resistance to stress. In this situation these types of approaches are temporary cover-ups that do not get at the root of the poor stress response.

To address the underlying triggers of HPA axis dysfunction, it is imperative to improve your nutritional status. A diet such as the Modified Mediterranean Diet discussed in Chapter 9 is extremely helpful. The benefits of the traditional Mediterranean diet are supported by a plethora of studies showing it reduces the risks of major diseases. The traditional diet revolves around vegetables, fruits, seafood, poultry, beans, herbs and spices, olive oil, nuts, moderate dairy, and limited red meat. There are plenty of free Mediterranean diet cookbooks available. I modify the Mediterranean diet to reduce wheat products, as they spike blood glucose and insulin and are a common food sensitivity. You should consume a limited amount of caffeine (one to two cups of coffee a day, or preferably green tea) as well as restrict simple sugar intake (less than 25 grams daily).

Stress reduction techniques, such as prayer, meditation, neurofeedback, and counseling, are also helpful. These approaches are often needed to address the deepest level of poor stress adaptation. Individual preferences to stress reduction techniques vary greatly, so focus on those you will be consistent with.

Regular exercise is important but needs to be light enough for you to recover adequately. The length and intensity vary depending on the individual. However, consistency is very important for HPA axis balancing.

Adequate quality sleep is essential. For most people, this means seven to eight hours. Sleep disorders like insomnia or apnea, if present, must be treated. Chapter 8 offers additional recommendations for insomnia.

Take HPA Axis–Balancing Supplements

I often have patients take an adrenal formula that contains a combination of adaptogenic herbs that work to balance the HPA axis and improve adrenal hormone balance. My favorite adaptogenic herbs include rhodiola rosea, ashwagandha, and eleutherococcus (Siberian ginseng). These herbs, along with nutrients such as B vitamins and vitamin C, are effective in helping people reestablish adrenal balance. And remember, the better your adrenal health, the better your gut health will be.

The European Medicines Agency (EMA) defines herbal adaptogens as follows: "Adaptogenic substances are stated to have the capacity to normalize body functions and strengthen systems compromised by stress. They are reported to have a protective effect on health against a wide variety of environmental assaults and emotional conditions."[6] The EMA also notes that adaptogens are virtually nontoxic to the user.

The two top herbal adaptogens I use are ashwagandha and rhodiola rosea. Ashwagandha has a long history of use in Ayurvedic medicine. There are several human studies published concerning its beneficial effects as an adaptogen. Ashwagandha extract has been studied in people with a history of chronic stress to improve their resistance to stress and quality of life scores based on a variety of questionnaires.[7] Perceived stress by the participants was reduced by 44 percent. In addition, after 60 days, serum cortisol levels were reduced by 27.9 percent from baseline compared to 7.9 percent of those in the placebo group. One other study worth mentioning is a double-blind, placebo-controlled trial, which found that 125 to 250 mg of ashwagandha extract taken twice daily led to a 79 percent reduction in fatigue as well as improvements in ratings of stress, anxiety, irritability, inability to concentrate, and forgetfulness.[8] These factors did not improve in the placebo group. Serum cortisol levels also decreased by 24.2 percent and DHEA levels improved by 32.2 percent for those taking ashwagandha extract. It should be noted that DHEA works to balance cortisol.

Ashwagandha is well tolerated. The recommended dose is 250 to 500 mg daily of a standardized extract.

Rhodiola is a medicinal plant that has had almost 200 studies published on its chemistry and clinical use. It has a long history of use in Siberian and Russian medicine as an adaptogen. It is also an effective antioxidant that protects the brain and nervous system from free radical damage. Rhodiola has been shown to increase physical work capacity and shorten recovery time between bouts of high-intensity exercise.

Recent research shows that rhodiola rosea has "anti-aging, anti-inflammation, immunostimulating, DNA repair, and anti-cancer effects in different model systems."[9] Moreover, the *International Journal of Psychiatry in Clinical Practice* revealed that Rhodiola rosea extract has the beneficial actions of "providing both physical and psychological symptom relief, normalising stress hormone levels and increasing energy."[10]

Rhodiola has multiple effects in the body, including effects on neurotransmitter production in the brain and balancing effects on the HPA axis.

Side effects are uncommon. The recommended dose is 200 to 300 mg of a standardized product containing 3 percent rosavins.

Additional Adrenal Supplements

Many nutrients support adrenal gland function. A good strategy is to include a high-potency multivitamin and mineral formulation and then include additional nutrients that have human/ animal studies for supporting adrenal function.

Additional recommendations include vitamin C (1000 to 2000 mg), B complex vitamins (follow directions on the label), pantothenic acid (100 to 250 mg), and magnesium (250 to 500 mg).

Adrenal Hormone Replacement

For patients who have more severe symptoms and lab testing that shows a deficiency of adrenal hormones, supplementing hormones such as DHEA, pregnenolone, and in limited cases, cortisol can be beneficial. DHEA and pregnenolone are available over the counter. Keep in mind that although they have direct effects on tissues, they also function as precursor hormones. For example, pregnenolone is a precursor to progesterone and DHEA, while DHEA is a precursor to testosterone and estrogen. These hormones should be used only under the guidance of a doctor.

WORKING WITH YOUR GENES

If you have been prone to anxiety and depression most of your life—and especially if it runs in your family—then you may have genetic predispositions to neurotransmitter imbalances. Are you familiar with a common genetic variation known as methylenetetrahydrofolate reductase (MTHFR) that makes people susceptible to depression? Studies show that a significant percent of the population have a variation in this gene, which controls an enzyme in all our cells that is involved in methylation, a chemical process that adds a carbon and three hydrogens onto other chemicals for life-sustaining processes such as producing energy, allowing our DNA to work, making hormones, detoxification, and making neurotransmitters. When you have inherited one or two variations or bad copies, then the enzyme it makes, known as methylenetetrahydrofolate reductase, functions at a slower rate and you can have certain health problems. Research reveals that people with these variations in the MTHFR genes known as C677T and A1298C are more likely to have psychiatric diseases like depression. For example, a meta-analysis involving 26 published studies concerning MTHFR polymorphism demonstrated "an obvious association of MTHFR C677T polymorphism with increased risk of depression."[11] This association was strongest in Asian populations.

When you have these MTHFR genetic variations, you cannot metabolize folic acid properly. Most people are surprised to find that folic acid is a synthetic or man-made B vitamin that you do not find in food. It's often used in supplements since it's cheap and does not degrade rapidly. The preferred form, known as folate or methylfolate, is the natural form found in foods such as spinach, dark green leafy vegetables, beans, nuts, peas, seafood, eggs, poultry, meat, and grains. You can also get folate or methylfolate in high-quality supplements. Your body uses folate for the MTHFR enzyme to work properly in many ways, including making neurotransmitters such as serotonin. This is why folate supplementation can help people with depression, and especially when used with active B_{12} such as methylcobalamin.

If you are prone to anxiety, you may have inherited variations with the catechol-O-methyltransferase (COMT) gene. This gene codes for the enzyme COMT, which is involved in the breakdown of stress chemicals in the body known as catecholamines (dopamine, norepinephrine, epinephrine). You can see how higher levels of these catecholamines lead to feelings of anxiety for some people. Support with magnesium, B complex, and molybdenum can be helpful. Work with a doctor knowledgeable in nutritional therapies for epigenetic support.

THE DIAPHRAGM DELIGHT

The diaphragm is located between the chest and abdominal cavity, and it is the major muscle of breathing. This dome-shaped muscle contracts and flattens when we take a breath in, which provides more height in the thoracic cavity, allowing more air to come in with increased lung volume. With expiration, the diaphragm relaxes. Interestingly, the diaphragm has a massaging effect on the organs below it (including the digestive organs) when we take in a deep breath.

There has been a lot of research demonstrating that slow and deep diaphragmatic breathing has beneficial effects on the brain and body. This technique involves taking in slow, deep breaths using the diaphragm muscle and minimum movement of the chest. One recommendation is to sit up straight (or lay flat), take slow deep breathes in through the nose and out through the mouth, and with one hand on your abdomen feel the abdomen move in and out instead of focusing on the chest.

Diaphragmatic breathing has a modulating effect on the nervous system and affects the respiratory, brain, cardiovascular, and gastrointestinal systems.[12] It has the following benefits:

- improves core muscle stability
- slows rate of breathing so you conserve energy
- provides a relaxing effect and lowers the stress hormone cortisol
- increases venous blood return to heart
- improves respiratory capacity
- lowers blood pressure
- helps with the symptoms of post-traumatic stress disorder
- improves ability to tolerate intense exercise
- lowers chance of injuries[13]

There are several videos, apps, and wearable devices on the market you can use to help monitor your diaphragmatic breathing.

FASTING

Many people feel less stressed and more rejuvenated after fasting. You may find fasting helps your body with the effects of stress. In Chapter 4 I discussed the benefits of fasting to allow your gut to heal. It gives the digestive organs and tract a break from metabolic work and gives the stem cells the opportunity for gut healing, as old cells are replaced with new—a process called autophagy.

Moreover, research has demonstrated that fasting reduces body inflammation, body weight, insulin resistance, blood pressure, and provides other benefits such as clarity of mind.[14]

Fasting may become a necessary medical therapy for most people, given the environmental toxin burden facing the United States and other countries around the world. For example, the Natural Resources Defense Council reported that there are 80,000 chemicals currently being used in the United States, and most of them have not been adequately tested for human health safety.[15]

There are many types of fasts that range from water only and juice only to intermittent fasting. The most practical for most people is intermittent fasting, which involves limiting the amount of hours one eats in a day. When you go without food for several hours (water not included), your body will rely on burning fat for energy. One common technique is to eat during an eight-hour window each day or several days a week. Another technique is the 5:2 approach, where you eat a healthy diet five days a week without time restriction, and then eat a low-calorie diet, such as 500 calories, for two days a week. Other people experienced in fasting may have water only one day a week or for several days one to two times a year.

One interesting modification with fasting is combining intermittent fasting with a Mediterranean diet (as given in Chapter 9). According to an article in the *Journal of the American College of Cardiology*, the combination of intermittent fasting (8 to 12 hours) along with a Pesco-Mediterranean diet (wherein you consume fish instead of other animal products) is the ideal cardioprotective diet.[16]

Do not try fasting if you are pregnant or breastfeeding. It also can be problematic for people with type 1 diabetes, children, teens, people who are underweight, and those with a history of eating disorders, and in these cases should only be used under a doctor's guidance.

STRESS FIGHTERS: SLEEP AND EXERCISE

I cannot emphasize the importance of good-quality sleep and exercise enough when it comes to detoxing from stress. Sleep is the time when the brain and body regenerate. For example, researchers have discovered an entirely new organ called the *glymphatic system*. The glymphatic system is a vascular network that includes lymphatics that remove waste products from the brain. According to *Brain Sciences*, the glymphatic system is constantly filtering toxins from the brain, but this mainly occurs during the sleep cycle.[17] However, when we are awake, the glymphatic detoxification is disengaged by about 90 percent. Interestingly, the glymphatic system removes the proteins (amyloid-beta and tau) that are associated with Alzheimer's disease and brain degradation. The journal also noted that lifestyle choices that negatively impact the glymphatic system include alcohol, lack of exercise, lack of omega-3 consumption, and stress. Benefits can be attained with intermittent fasting by improving the functioning of the glymphatic system. If you have trouble sleeping, see the section on insomnia in Chapter 8.

Exercise is fundamental to maintaining stress hormone balance, healthy immunity and inflammation control, and other factors that affect gut function. In *Frontiers in Nutrition*, researchers discussed the benefits of moderate exercise on intestinal permeability and the gut microbiota.[18] However, the same researchers found that excessive exercise, such as in overtraining, resulted in leaky gut, reduced gut mucus thickness, and possibly increased inflammation. Optimal exercise routines generally include regular forms of aerobic activity and non-aerobic (such as resistance training). Most people should be involved in some form of daily exercise. If you have health conditions that require specialized exercise, then consult with a trainer or sports-oriented doctor.

OTHER STRESS-REDUCING THERAPIES

There are several stress-reducing therapies that can alleviate the effects of stress and help your gut heal. These include those that relax and balance the muscoskeletal system, such as acupuncture, massage, and chiropractic. Also, neurofeedback and biofeedback can be used to balance the mind and nervous system. Work with reputable practitioners to receive these helpful therapies.

WHICH STRESS REDUCTION TECHNIQUES ARE BEST FOR YOU?

In a world of what can feel like unrelenting stress, it's important to detox from stress on a regular basis to ensure gut and whole-body health. There are numerous ways to reduce the effects of stress, such as prayer, meditation, stretching, yoga, exercise, humor and laughter, counseling, volunteering, neurofeedback/biofeedback, and many others. Research is demonstrating that these techniques can improve the health of gut microbiota. For example, a study published in *Frontiers in Cellular and Infection Microbiology* reported that mindfulness-based cognitive therapy (MBCT) improved gut microbiota balance.[19] Ultimately, techniques that work for you and that are healthy (for example, not excess alcohol consumption or recreational drugs) should be part of a regular routine.

Chapter 7

PROTOCOLS FOR TARGETING DIGESTIVE ISSUES

Larry, a 50-year-old lawyer, came to my office with concerns about the long-term effects of taking a PPI medication for his GERD (he'd been on it for two years at the time). He had tried to stop it in the past, but his GERD was very problematic, and his primary doctor told him he'd have to take a PPI for the rest of his life. I had him stop eating after 6:00 P.M., especially fatty or heavy meals. I also told him not to consume any alcohol until I had treated him for a few months. I put him on a powder before meals that had aloe, DGL, and glutamine as well as extracts of *Opuntia ficus-indica* and *Olea europaea* twice daily. I told him to take his PPI medication every other day starting in six weeks. He was able to do this without a relapse in his GERD. Next, I had him take his PPI every third day for six weeks and he was successful with this as well. Six months later, he continued to do well and to date has not had to use his PPI medication.

In the previous chapters you read about how to address your leaky gut and dysbiosis in general with diet, targeted supplements, and stress reduction. In this chapter I will drill down and focus on specific digestive issues and how they can be treated with these natural approaches. I will provide clinical insights to help you understand how to improve these conditions from an integrative or functional medicine perspective. While the core digestive treatment plan is helpful for all these ailments, I will also give you specialized strategies based on the scientific research and my clinic experience for additional help in treating each of these conditions. If you have health problems, make sure to check with your doctor first before starting new therapies.

My approach to treating leaky gut and dysbiosis is of course highly effective for digestive problems. Since my approach targets the digestive system, it makes for a great way to reestablish health with many common digestive problems. And as you have now learned, the healthier your digestive system, the healthier your body will become.

The following conditions are addressed in this chapter in alphabetical order:

- acid reflux (GERD)

- candida overgrowth

- constipation

- gallstones

- gastritis

- inflammatory bowel disease (Crohn's disease and ulcerative colitis)

- irritable bowel syndrome

- lactose intolerance

- small intestine bacterial overgrowth (SIBO)

- ulcers

ACID REFLUX (GERD)

Acid reflux, also referred to as acid indigestion, reflux, or heartburn, occurs when stomach acid flows upward to the esophagus. People feel a sensation of burning, pressure, or some type of discomfort in the upper middle abdomen region and chest. Approximately 60 million people in the U.S. experience acid reflux at least once monthly. Gastroesophageal reflux disease (GERD) is the progression to a more severe form of acid reflux where heartburn is more frequent at two or more times a week. Food and liquid from the stomach can move upward through the esophagus and into the mouth. In addition to a burning or uncomfortable sensation in the chest, you may experience symptoms after eating and lying down, the sensation of a lump in the throat, trouble swallowing, sore throat, coughing, asthma-like symptoms, increased saliva production, sour or acid liquid in the mouth (from regurgitation of food or liquids), nausea, and hoarseness. Between 20 to 28 percent of the U.S. population has GERD.

Acid reflux and GERD are more common in people who are of a higher weight, pregnant women, smokers, those who have a hiatal hernia, those who use of certain medications (e.g., non-steroidal anti-inflammatory drugs), and those who consume unhealthy foods.

The main issue with acid reflux and GERD is an abnormality of the lower esophageal sphincter (LES), which is not closing properly. The LES is the valve between the stomach and esophagus. Normally, when we swallow, the LES relaxes and allows food and liquid to flow into the stomach and then subsequently tightens again to keep the stomach content in the stomach. When the LES relaxes too much or weakens, it does not stop stomach acid from flowing up into the esophagus. Another factor can be problems with esophageal peristalsis (movement of food and liquid down the esophagus to the stomach). Carrying a high amount of body fat also puts pressure on the LES and stimulates it to stay open. Additional triggers for abnormal function of the LES include eating large meals at night; eating trigger foods, such as fried, fatty, or spicy foods; and consuming certain beverages like coffee and alcohol.

You should also consider spinal causes from the neck (cervical) and upper to mid back (thoracic), since nerve flow to the stomach and LES could be abnormal. Chiropractic and other holistic providers can assess spinal-related causes.

There is emerging evidence that gut dysbiosis is associated with GERD. Dysbiosis leads to increased inflammation of the stomach and esophagus. People with GERD also have a higher incidence of SIBO, which may predispose them to GERD and leaky gut syndrome. Therefore, managing and improving the gut microbiome is an important long-term approach to GERD. This brings up the topic of proton pump inhibitors (PPIs), such as dexlansoprazole (Dexilant), esomeprazole (Nexium), lansoprazole (Prevacid), omeprazole (Prilosec), pantoprazole (Protonix), and rabeprazole (Aciphex). PPIs are a common pharmaceutical treatment for GERD prescribed by doctors and also available over the counter. Approximately 58 million prescriptions are given each year in the United States. PPIs suppress stomach acid secretion but over time create gut dysbiosis and increased risk of SIBO. They are also associated with causing nutrient deficiencies, which may affect gut and body health. The normal recommended time period for PPI use is four to eight weeks. Many people are on PPIs for much longer than this, which can create other digestive and body health problems. Research published in *Neurogastroenterology & Motility* has shown that PPIs cause leaky gut in mice studies.[1] Treatment of GERD should include whole digestive health, including the microbiome throughout the gut as well as addressing leaky gut syndrome.

People with GERD should have their esophagus evaluated with endoscopy to make sure no damage has occurred and there are no precancerous or cancerous changes to the esophagus tissue. Fortunately, a high percentage of people with acid reflux or GERD respond well to the holistic treatments discussed in this section.

Treatment

Improvement in diet and weight balance is the primary approach to help most people with acid reflux and GERD. Moderate to severe cases often benefit from the additional use of supplements described in this section. If you have been taking a medication for GERD long-term, such as a PPI, and want to follow a natural protocol instead of the drug, then it is best to have your doctor slowly lower the dose over time, while following the natural protocol below. There can be a rebound effect when stopping PPIs abruptly that can flare up GERD.

I had a review study published in the *Journal of Nutritional Health & Food Engineering*, in which I discussed the research on the dietary approach to helping GERD.[2] One of the studies I reviewed included 85 patients treated with PPIs, while 88 additional patients followed a Mediterranean-style diet (restricting animal products more than typical) and drank alkaline water. Both groups avoided foods known to commonly trigger acid reflux, such as coffee, tea, soda, greasy and fatty foods, chocolate, spicy foods, and alcohol. Researchers found that of those who made the diet changes, 62.6 percent showed a clinically meaningful improvement, while of those taking PPIs, 54.1 percent showed a clinically meaningful improvement. The reduction in reflux symptom index also was significantly better in the diet group (39.8 percent) than in the PPI group (27.2 percent). A different study in *Diseases of the Esophagus* found the protective effects against GERD for the Mediterranean diet were related to the diet as a whole, not any single component.[3]

Try to consume the last meal of the day earlier in the evening or late afternoon—I recommend eating dinner at least three hours before bedtime. I have seen many patients experience good improvement in GERD just by following this approach. If you do eat later in the evening, make sure the meal is light and not fatty. If you are prone to GERD, avoid caffeine and alcohol in the evening. Since dysbiosis is so common with GERD, make sure to regularly consume prebiotic and probiotic foods in Chapter 9 to optimize your microbiome.

Sleeping position can also help GERD. Some people experience improvements by sleeping on their left side. Using adjustable beds where the top of the bed is propped up by at least six inches or using special slanted whole-body pillows can be helpful. If you have sleep problems, have your doctor test you for sleep apnea as this condition is also linked to GERD.

Supplement with aloe, DGL, and glutamine, as I discussed in Chapter 5. Out of these three natural supplements, the most important is aloe and DGL. These supplements reduce inflammation of the esophagus, stomach, and GI tract, and they stimulate the production of the protective mucin layer of the stomach.

Supplement with the combination of extracts of *Opuntia ficus-indica* and *Olea europaea*, known as Mucosave™ FG. A randomized double-blind placebo-controlled study investigated the effect of these two extracts with 60 participants taking Mucosave™ FG (400 mg) and 40 participants taking a placebo.[4] Participants filled out digestive-related questionnaires before the start of the study and after four and eight weeks, as well as a daily diary of how they felt. Those receiving the Mucosave™ FG had a significant improvement in their scores for gastrointestinal discomfort and GERD, including reflux, abdominal pain, belching, pressure in the chest, food back in mouth (regurgitation), and gurgling of the abdomen. Benefits were noted from the first day of supplementation.

Supplement with digestive enzymes, especially if you have food sensitivities, are under chronic stress, are consuming large meals, or are eating late at night. Supplement 3 mg of melatonin at bedtime, which has been shown to help treat GERD. Melatonin is a hormone produced in the brain (pineal gland) as well as by cells in the gut. It improves circulation to the mucosa of the gut as well as mucosal growth and repair, reduces inflammation, and activates hormones and messengers that activate closure of the LES.[5] A study found that 3 mg of melatonin was effective by itself or in combination with omeprazole for treating GERD.[6] The same study found melatonin improved the activity of LES.

Supplement probiotics with human-studied strains. A review of 13 studies containing different *Lactobacillus* and *Bifidobacterium* strains found that the majority of research reported benefits for GERD.[7]

CANDIDA OVERGROWTH

Candida is a type of fungus, and more specifically a type of yeast, that lives in the digestive tract as a commensal organism and is considered a part of the microbiome. *Candida* yeast is opportunistic, and when given the right environment, it can flourish and become pathogenic in the digestive tract, vaginal and urinary tract, and in severe cases in the immunocompromised bloodstream.

The industrialized Western diet and the use of antibiotics are thought to be the reasons why the Western population is colonized by *Candida albicans* more than in other societies.[8] Along the same lines, excessive refined sugar promotes the overgrowth of fungi like *Candida albicans* that can cause a leaky gut.[9] Moreover, *Candida albicans* is known to create biofilms that make it difficult for the immune system to remove it. Biofilms are substances secreted by microbes such as Candida that adhere to the gut and make it more difficult for the immune system to penetrate them.

Many conventional medicine practitioners believe that *Candida* is only a problem in limited cases, such as in temporary thrush of the mouth after antibiotics, or in immunocompromised individuals having systemic infections with *Candida*. It is interesting to note that medical journals like *Tissue Barriers* state that damage to the intestinal mucosal barrier and dysbiosis are major risk factors for *Candida albicans* to become a life-threatening infection that spreads into the bloodstream and throughout the body.[10]

However, many people have overgrowth of *Candida* that compromises their digestive and gut health. While they usually do not have life-threatening illnesses, a variety of symptoms, such as headaches, skin rashes, irritable bowel syndrome, bloating, focus problems, and other issues, may result from *Candida* overgrowth. Holistic doctors often assess *Candida* status with stool, urine, or blood tests.

Treatment

Dietary changes that prevent the feeding of yeast through a low/simple-carbohydrate diet with moderate healthy fat and protein are important. This could include a paleo diet, a modified ketogenic diet, and the Modified Mediterranean Diet in Chapter 9. Excellent meal-planning books by Doug Kaufmann, an expert in *Candida*, are available. It is also important to avoid alcohol consumption, which feeds yeast. Do consume prebiotic and probiotic foods as given in Chapter 9 to provide friendly flora that naturally crowd out yeast and reestablish microbiome balance, and consider supplementing with prebiotics and probiotics.

Supplement natural antifungal agents, such as oregano oil, garlic, grapefruit seed extract, Pau d'arco, and caprylic acid. *Candida* combination products are readily available. Supplement milk thistle (250 mg to 500 mg) with meals to support detoxification during antifungal therapy.

Supplement L-glutathione between meals to support detoxification during antifungal therapy (250 mg twice daily).

Consider antifungal medications for a short course of treatment if you have a severe case of fungal overgrowth. Examples include Nystatin, Fluconazole, and others.

Peter, a 61-year-old salesmen, had been dealing with candida issues for several years. When he followed a low-sugar diet and took anti-candida supplements or antifungal medications, his candida-related symptoms, such as bloating, fatigue, brain fog, and sinusitis, improved. However, within three to four months, his *Candida* symptoms would return, and testing would show Candida activity. After following my leaky gut and dysbiosis corrective program for four months, Peter did not have any more relapses. It has now been three years since my treatment, and he continues to do well and does not require *Candida* treatment.

CONSTIPATION

Constipation refers to infrequent bowel movements or difficulty passing stools that lasts for several weeks or longer. Conventional medicine teaches that a frequency of passing less than three bowel movements a week is constipation. While this may be a working medical definition, it certainly is not considered optimal within integrative and naturopathic medicine. One to three complete bowel movements per day is considered by many digestive experts to be optimal.

There are various causes of constipation, such as medical issues causing physical blockages of the digestive tract, abnormal nerve function of the GI tract, muscular problems of the pelvic muscles involved in passage of stool, eating disorders, and hormonal issues like hypothyroidism or diabetes. The main causes of chronic constipation include a lack of fiber in the diet, lack of water, not enough exercise, neurotransmitter and hormone imbalance, and the use of certain medications (e.g., opioids). Some of the complications of chronic constipation include hemorrhoids, anal fissures (small tears in the anus), inability to expel stool (fecal impaction), and rectal prolapse.

According to a study published in the *World Journal of Clinical Cases*, when stool elimination is delayed in the gut, it adversely affects the gut microbiome and results in increased mucus production as the body compensates with trying to eliminate stool.[11] Several studies have demonstrated a connection between gut dysbiosis and constipation.[12] Stool consistency is associated with the diversity of gut microbiota and composition.[13] In the SIBO section in this chapter, I discuss how the methane type is related to constipation. In addition, adults with constipation have significantly lower amounts of the flora *Bifidobacteria* and *Lactobacilli* and increased bacteroidetes in stool samples compared to control subjects.[14]

Treatment

The cornerstone of treatment for chronic constipation is the increased consumption of water and fiber. Most people with constipation will improve by focusing on these two dietary requirements.

Increasing water intake between 50 to 80 ounces daily is helpful for some people with constipation. However, not everyone with chronic constipation will respond to increasing their amount of water. Increased water, higher fiber diet or supplements, and exercise should be the first line of approach to chronic constipation.

According to the Academy of Nutrition and Dietetics, only 5 percent of the U.S. adult population achieve an adequate intake of fiber.[15] For women this amount is 25 grams, and for men it is 38 grams. When looking at labels, 2.5 grams per serving is considered a "good source," while 5 grams per serving is an "excellent source." The key to increasing fiber intake is consuming plant foods that contain indigestive carbohydrates and lignins (found in many whole plant foods—whole grains, nuts and seeds, legumes, and so on). Good sources include whole grains (caution for those with gluten allergy or sensitivity), vegetables, fruits, legumes, and nuts. Keep in mind that the processing of foods reduces fiber content. Most grains people consume, such as breads and pastas, are refined. There is also insoluble fiber in beans, oat bran, fruits, and vegetables that does not significantly increase fecal bulk but has other benefits such as blood sugar regulation and satiety.

Increased fiber helps bowel movements by increasing stool bulk, increasing stool frequency, and reducing stool transit time through the intestines. Fiber also retains water (especially soluble fiber) and when fermented in the digestive tract the resulting bacteria increase stool mass. Moreover, fiber helps in weight balance and provides a full feeling to reduce appetite. Increased fiber in the diet also reduces the risk of certain diseases, such as cardiovascular diseases, type 2 diabetes, and certain cancers.

HIGH-FIBER FOODS

Following are examples of food categories and their fiber intake (data sourced from the U.S. Department of Agriculture Food-Data Central, Dietary Guidelines for Americans, and Academy of Nutrition and Dietetics):[16]

Fruits

Apple with skin (large), 5.4 grams
Pear with skin (medium), 5.5 grams
Raspberries (½ cup), 4.0 grams
Strawberries (1 cup sliced), 3.3 grams
Orange, 3.1 grams

Vegetables

Split peas, cooked (½ cup), 8.1 grams
Lentils, cooked (½ cup), 7.8 grams
Kidney beans, canned (½ cup), 5.5 grams
Artichoke, cooked (½ cup), 4.8 grams
Navy beans, cooked (½ cup), 4.8 grams
Lima beans, cooked (½ cup), 4.6 grams
Sweet potato, no skin (½ cup), 4.1 grams
Pinto beans, cooked (½ cup), 3.6 grams
Black beans, cooked (½ cup), 3.75 grams
Green peas, canned (½ cup), 3.5 grams
Potato, baked, skin on (1 medium), 3.3 grams
Carrots, raw (8 baby carrots), 2.5 grams
Cauliflower, cooked (1 cup), 2.45 grams
Spinach, cooked (½ cup), 2.2 grams
Broccoli, raw (½ cup), 1.1 grams
Lettuce, iceberg (1 cup, shredded), 0.9 grams

Grains

Raisin Bran (1 cup), 7.4 grams
Shredded Wheat (2 biscuits), 5.5 grams
Rice, brown, cooked (1 cup), 3.5 grams
Barley, pearled, cooked (½ cup), 3.0 grams
Oatmeal, cooked (¾ cup), 3.0 grams
Bread, whole wheat (1 slice), 1.9 grams

Rye crispbread (1 wafer), 1.6 grams
Tortillas, whole wheat (1 ounce), 2.8 grams

Nuts and Seeds
Almonds (¼ cup), 4.5 grams
Walnuts (¼ cup, pieces), 2.0 grams
Pumpkin seeds (¼ cup), 1.935 grams
Sunflower seeds (¼ cup), 3.275 grams
Pistachio nuts (¼ cup), 3.25 grams

An additional consideration is the potential role of food sensitivities for chronic constipation. Some people find the identification and restriction of food sensitivities can be helpful in alleviating this condition. One of the common food sensitivities for chronic constipation is cow's milk products.

Make sure to regularly consume the prebiotic and probiotic foods in Chapter 9 to optimize your microbiome and promote regularity. Supplement a probiotic with human-studied strains.

Supplement with psyllium seed fiber if you are having trouble getting enough fiber in your diet. Take one teaspoon (5 grams of fiber) with 10 ounces of water two to three times daily. Gradually increase your dose. Psyllium is also available in capsule form.

Supplement triphala, composed of the fruits of *Terminalia chebula* (black myrobalan), *Terminalia bellerica* (bastard myrobalan) and *Phyllantus emblica* (Indian gooseberry). The journal *Chinese Medicine* reported that triphala can be used long-term to improve bowel movements.[17] Unlike laxatives it does not have a stimulating effect on the bowels but rather a regulatory effect. A typical dose is 500 to 1000 mg daily of the capsule or tablet form.

Regular exercise and stress-reduction techniques as discussed in Chapter 6 can also be helpful for chronic constipation.

GALLSTONES

The number of people in the United States with gallstones is growing, with up to 20 percent suffering from this condition.[18] It is the most common digestive condition causing hospitalization. Gallstones occur in the gallbladder, a pear-shaped organ below the liver. The function of the gallbladder is to receive bile from the liver and then store and release bile into the small intestine to support fat digestion. The main type of gallstone is formed from a supersaturation of cholesterol and is usually responsible for blocking the ducts. The other form is pigment stones, which are made of bilirubin and calcium complexes. Black pigment stones typically stay in the gallbladder.

If small enough, gallstones may not cause symptoms. However, a gallstone lodged in a duct can cause pain in the upper right abdomen, center of abdomen, between the shoulder blades, and in the right shoulder, and it can cause nausea and vomiting.

People at risk for gallstones include women (with a higher risk during pregnancy or when using birth control pills and certain forms of hormone replacement); those with a family history of gallstones; and those with liver cirrhosis, infection of the bile ducts, hemolytic anemias, Crohn's disease, high triglyceride levels, low HDL cholesterol, insulin resistance and diabetes, obesity, and rapid weight loss.

Emerging evidence has shown that the gut microbiome plays a role in the risk of gallstone disease.[19] The increased risk arises due to the gut microbiota playing a role in bile acid metabolism. Bile acids are involved in fat digestion by emulsifying and solubilizing fats, and they prevent the saturation of cholesterol in the formation of the most common gallstones. The biliary and gut microbiota play a role in lipid and cholesterol metabolism. In addition, bile acids are influenced by bacteria from the mouth (saliva) and bacteria that migrate from the small intestine. The bacteria that affects the stomach, *Helicobacter pylori*, is also known to be a contributor to cholesterol gallstone formation. Researchers have found that the diversity of the microbiome of the gut and biliary tract are reduced and varied in people with gallstone disease.

Treatment

Asymptomatic gallstones can be treated with diet, bile salt therapy, and lithotripsy (shockwaves that break the stones down, so they pass). Gallbladder removal (cholecystectomy) may be necessary when there is gallbladder pain or infection. Gallstones lodged in a duct can be removed with procedures that do not require gallbladder removal.

If you have gallstones, you'll want to consume a reduced-fat diet. This does not mean that you need to avoid all fat, especially healthy fats. You can follow the Modified Mediterranean Diet in Chapter 9. You can also take lipase enzymes, which digest fats when taken with meals. Bile salts emulsify and digest fats and reduce saturation of cholesterol in bile, and you can take as directed on the label. Also supplement prebiotics and probiotics to balance the microbiome.

GASTRITIS

Gastritis refers to inflammation of the stomach lining. Symptoms can include pain (burning or gnawing) in the upper abdomen, nausea, vomiting, and a sensation of fullness in the upper abdomen. Some people have gastritis without signs and symptoms. Causes of gastritis include a bacterial infection known as Helicobacter pylori and other infectious agents, NSAIDs (such as aspirin, ibuprofen, and other medications), stress, diet, and alcohol.

Treatment

The holistic treatment of gastritis is the same as for acid reflux, except that the infectious bacteria Helicobacter pylori (H. pylori) needs to be treated if present. The conventional treatment of H. pylori includes antibiotics, PPI, and sometimes bismuth. Antibiotic resistance and recurrent infection are problematic for H. pylori. This makes natural approaches important in the treatment of this bacterial infection.

I have found H. pylori can be treated effectively in many cases with natural therapies, such as mastic gum, DGL, zinc carnosine, and probiotics. A study found that mastic gum at the dose of 350 mg to 1005 grams three times daily could eradicate H. pylori for some people suffering from infection.[20] Research has also demonstrated that mastic gum significantly improves symptoms for people with dyspepsia (indigestion), including stomach pain.[21]

Licorice root (DGL) has been shown to have anti-H. pylori effects and heals the gut mucosa. DGL (a type of licorice extract readily available) was shown to be effective in several human studies for the treatment of stomach and small intestine issues. One study found DGL to be comparable to the drug cimetidine (Tagamet) in treating ulcers.[22] DGL is best taken before meals in chewable tablet (760 to 1520 mg) or powder form.

Zinc carnosine is used to treat H. pylori and to heal ulcers. A paper in *Nutrients* demonstrated the anti–H. pylori effects of zinc carnosine.[23] In addition, the same review showed that zinc carnosine combined with conventional drug treatment is more effective than drug treatment only for the treatment of H. pylori. A typical dose is 150 mg twice daily with meals.

Probiotics, especially *Lactobacillus* species, have been shown to have anti–*H. pylori* activity. *Lactobacillus* reduces gastritis, promotes the formation of the stomach mucus layer, and improves the effectiveness of antibiotics for *H. pylori* treatment.[24] Additional research has shown probiotics make it more difficult for *H. pylori* to colonize the stomach lining, form compounds that kill bacteria, modulate the immune response and reduce stomach inflammation, and improve immune response with antibodies.[25] However, probiotics alone have not been shown to eradicate H. pylori, so they should be used with other natural agents and if needed, along with antibiotics.

INFLAMMATORY BOWEL DISEASE (CROHN'S DISEASE AND ULCERATIVE COLITIS)

The term *inflammatory bowel disease (IBD)* refers to chronic inflammation of the lining of the digestive tract. There are two diseases within this category: Crohn's disease and ulcerative colitis.

Crohn's disease may involve the deeper layers of the gastrointestinal tract and mainly affects the small intestine and large intestine. However, Crohn's disease can affect the GI tract from the mouth to the anus. Symptoms can include abdominal pain and cramping, diarrhea, fever, weight loss, blood in stool, mouth sores, and anemia. Other areas of the body outside of the digestive system can be affected as well. We do not know exactly why people develop Crohn's disease, but certainly diet, stress, family history, smoking, and nonsteroidal anti-inflammatory medications are risk factors. In addition, food sensitivities and undiagnosed infections may play a role for some individuals. As I discussed earlier in the book, leaky gut is a common problem with Crohn's disease.

Ulcerative colitis (UC) involves inflammation of the colon and sometimes rectum. Symptoms can include diarrhea (may contain pus or blood), rectal bleeding and or pain, abdominal cramping and pain, urge to defecate, fatigue, fever, and weight loss.

Medically speaking the exact cause of UC is unknown. The condition is more common in people who have a family history of UC. Known risk factors include age (often but not always starts before the age of 30) and race (elevated risk in white people and people of Ashkenazi Jewish descent). Testing for Crohn's disease and UC involves stool analysis, colonoscopy, and imaging studies.

Treatment

Many people with IBD find they have better symptom control on a carbohydrate-restricted diet. However, the response to this type of diet varies. Also, reactivity to gluten, dairy, and sugar products is quite common. I recommend reviewing the dietary approach for Irritable Bowel Syndrome and consider the Modified Mediterranean Diet in Chapter 9. Also, the Specific Carbohdyrate Diet (SCD) can be very effective for IBD. This diet is grain-free and low in sugar and lactose.[26] Also, make sure to regularly consume prebiotic and probiotic foods to optimize your microbiome.

Since IBD can be very serious, it is important to work with doctors and nutritionists trained in clinical nutrition. Food sensitivity testing, stool analysis, and intestinal permeability testing and monitoring can be helpful.

Consider taking the following supplements:

- Prebiotics and probiotics to establish microbiome balance

- Turmeric and ginger with meals to reduce inflammation

- High-potency fish oil to reduce inflammation with omega-3s

- Digestive enzymes to reduce colon inflammation

- Bitters or betaine hydrochloride with meals to improve digestion

Consult with an integrative doctor on the use of the medication low-dose naltrexone (LDN) for IBD.

IRRITABLE BOWEL SYNDROME

Irritable bowel syndrome (IBS) is the most common digestive ailment that people consult with a doctor about. It is estimated to affect 10 to 15 percent of the adult population and is more common in females. IBS also occurs in children and adolescents. Typical symptoms include abdominal pain, gas, stool mucus, bloating, diarrhea, constipation, or alternating constipation and diarrhea.

People with IBS often experience other conditions such as fibromyalgia, chronic fatigue syndrome, and chronic pelvic pain. There are three main types of IBS, which include:

- IBS with constipation (IBS-C)
- IBS with diarrhea (IBS-D)
- IBS mixed type (IBS-M)

There are different root causes for IBS. Research has shown that genetics (it's more common if a family member has IBS), stressful life events, and infection of your digestive tract can all play a role. At a deeper level there is more going on. As I've discussed in the book, leaky gut and dysbiosis are common issues with IBS and need to be addressed for multiple reasons.

When you have leaky gut, it causes an inflammatory response in the small intestine, which can cause digestive symptoms. Also, leaky gut contributes to food sensitivities or intolerances, which are common for people with IBS. Moreover, problems with dysbiosis lead to inflammation in the digestive tract as well as fermentation and gas production. And there is the common problem of undiagnosed chronic infections in the gut. Bacterial overgrowth in the small intestine (SIBO) is a common cause of IBS. This is why testing, such as stool analysis and breath testing for SIBO, can be helpful. Research has found that people with IBS commonly have SIBO.[28] Many people with IBS have problems with fungal overgrowth in the gut, particularly *Candida albicans*. As I discussed earlier in the book, fungi and yeast such as *Candida* are a normal part of the flora (mycobiome), but due to diet, antibiotic use, and other factors, the *Candida* can overgrow. Overgrowth of *Candida* contributes to gas, bloating, loose stool, and abdominal cramping. There can be other infectious agents in the gut causing problems, such as parasitic or bacterial infections. (See also "Candida Overgrowth" on page 129 and "Small Intestine Bacterial Overgrowth (SIBO)" on page 144 in this chapter.)

There can be a connection between IBS and other digestive problems. We know that people with IBS are more likely to experience dyspepsia (indigestion) and gastroesophageal reflux disease (acid reflux). (See also "Acid Reflux [GERD]" on page 125 in this chapter.)

Stress is a root cause or trigger of IBS for some people. People with IBS are more likely to have problems with mental conditions, such as anxiety, depression, and somatic disorder (anxiety about physical symptoms). If you notice your IBS flares up when under stress (mental, emotional, or physical), then it is important to follow the recommendations in Chapter 6. (See also "Anxiety" on page 156 and "Depression" on page 161 in Chapter 8.)

Another factor in treating IBS is the role of food sensitivities. People with IBS frequently have intolerances to certain foods. Most often these food reactions are delayed, which can make it harder to pinpoint the offending foods. You can follow a hypoallergenic diet by eliminating common food sensitivities—such as dairy, gluten, corn, soy, citrus, and peanuts—for two to four weeks and see if there is a reduction in gut symptoms. If so, you can reintroduce a different food every three to five days to see which foods are problematic. From there you can restrict or rotate those food sensitivities. Another technique would be to pick a common food sensitivity group (for example, dairy) and avoid that food group only for a week and see if there is improvement. You could test one food every week or so to figure out any potential sensitivities. You can also have food sensitivity blood testing done through a lab. Food antibody tests are available, which can help take the guesswork out of identifying food sensitivities. If you have more than five food sensitivities, or if you seem to be developing food sensitivities over time, then be suspicious of leaky gut syndrome and take the appropriate steps in healing your gut to reverse the overactive immune response to foods.

TESTING FOR COMMON CAUSES OF IBS

- Stool test for evaluating microbiome and dysbiosis, infectious agents (*Candida*, parasites, etc.), leaky gut (zonulin), digestive enzyme levels, and how food is being broken down and absorbed (e.g., excess fat in stool)
- Breath test for small intestine bacterial overgrowth (SIBO)
- Elimination diet or blood antibody tests for food sensitivities
- Evaluation by a practitioner for how you cope with stress

Treatment

Consume a healthy diet that restricts fast foods and focuses on unprocessed foods. The Modified Mediterranean Diet in Chapter 9 is dairy and gluten free, which works well for many people with IBS. Make sure to regularly consume the prebiotic and probiotic foods in Chapter 9 to optimize your microbiome. Try increasing the amount of fiber in your diet gradually over time. You may find that some vegetables need to be lightly cooked or steamed until your digestion has improved.

Supplement with aloe, glutamine, DGL, a probiotic, and digestive enzymes or bitters with meals. Supplement with enteric-coated peppermint oil before meals, if you are having a flare-up of IBS.

Exercise regularly (30 to 60 minutes daily), and make sure your spinal alignment is correct to ensure proper nerve and blood flow to the digestive system. Incorporate stress-reduction techniques and consider counseling if you have trouble controlling the effects of stress. Acupuncture can also help with stress. Make sure to get enough sleep.

Anna, a 34-year-old accountant, had suffered from IBS with diarrhea intermittently for 15 years. She had improvement with a very restricted diet, but she had trouble maintaining a healthy weight and had high stress due to limited food choices, so she gave up on restricting her foods. My testing showed leaky gut as well as SIBO. She followed my protocol for leaky gut as well as for SIBO for three months. She noticed improvement in her symptoms within seven days, including less bloating and abdominal cramping. She found that over the next two months she rarely had loose stool, unless she had a high amount of cow's milk. To resolve this problem, she took enzymes on the occasions she had dairy and remains virtually symptom-free three years later.

LACTOSE INTOLERANCE

Lactose intolerance (LI) refers to the inability to digest the milk sugar lactose. The small intestine does not produce enough of the enzyme lactase. Common symptoms include gas, diarrhea, bloating, abdominal pain, and nausea. Approximately 50 to 90 percent of adult populations in African, Asian, and South American countries have LI, whereas 5 to 15 percent of people in European and North American countries have LI.

As people age, the small intestine generally produces less lactase. Genetics also play a role in lactose intolerance. In addition, illnesses and damage to the small intestine, celiac disease, SIBO, and Crohn's disease can be a cause. There are different tests your doctor can order to diagnose LI. However, for many people, LI is obvious from the symptoms they have after consuming milk and milk products.

Treatment

Those with LI should restrict or avoid milk products that cause problems. Cheeses and yogurt have lower levels of lactose and may be tolerated. Lactose-free and lactose-reduced milk and milk products are available. However, there are many dairy-free milks and milk products available now. Examples include coconut milk and yogurt, macadamia nut milk and yogurt, rice milk, almond milk, soy milk, and pea milk as well as cheeses that are dairy-free. The Modified Mediterranean Diet in Chapter 9 is dairy-free. Make sure to regularly consume the prebiotic and probiotic foods in Chapter 9 to optimize your microbiome involved in lactose breakdown.

Supplement with a lactase enzyme if you want to consume lactose-containing foods. These enzymes are available over the counter. In addition, there are enzyme formulas that contain lactase as well as additional enzymes that break down other sensitivity-provoking proteins in dairy products.

In addition to probiotic foods, you may want to supplement with probiotics, which improve the small intestine breakdown of lactase, decrease lactose concentration in fermented products, and increase the colonic fermentation of lactose.[29] Types of probiotic species shown to help LI include *Bifidobacterium animalis*, *Bifidobacterium longum*, *Lactobacillus reuteri*, and *Lactobacillus rhamnosus*.

SMALL INTESTINE BACTERIAL OVERGROWTH (SIBO)

Small intestine bacterial overgrowth (SIBO) has emerged as a common cause of abdominal bloating, pain, flatulence, loose stool, nausea, malabsorption, leaky gut, and low appetite. It is also a common trigger of IBS. With this condition there is the overgrowth of bacteria in the small intestine that do not normally inhabit this region. There are several different causes of SIBO:

- *Food poisoning* can damage the motor complex involved in peristalsis and impede the movement of food through GI tract. Bacteria from the colon then migrate to the small intestine.

- *Low stomach acid* allows bacteria to penetrate the digestive tract (stomach acid is a normal barrier to bacteria). The use of proton pump inhibitors (PPIs) is a known cause of SIBO.

- *Low bile flow* increases susceptibility to bacteria penetrating the digestive tract.

- *Low pancreatic enzyme output* (pancreatic insufficiency) impedes the digestion of food and the breakdown of bacteria in the small intestine. It is known that pancreatic insufficiency is associated with SIBO.

- *Abdominal surgeries* such as gastric bypass and others may cause SIBO. In addition, scar tissue and adhesions can impede small intestine activity.

- *Various medical conditions* (diabetes, celiac disease, diverticulosis, Crohn's disease, radiation therapy to the area, and others) can slow the passage of food through the small intestine and cause a buildup of bacteria.

Untreated SIBO increases the risk of leaky gut, vitamin deficiencies (A, D, K, E, B_{12}), and problems related to poor calcium absorption, such as osteoporosis and kidney stones.

The main testing method used to diagnose SIBO is a breath test, in which you collect a baseline breath test and then consume a sugar drink. Then more breath samples are collected to measure levels of hydrogen, methane, and hydrogen sulfide. These gases are formed when there is an overgrowth of bacteria. Elevated hydrogen produced by fermenting bacteria also fuels methane and hydrogen sulfide–producing organisms. Each of these gases correlate with a digestive condition:

- *Hydrogen:* loose stool or general SIBO symptoms

- *Methane:* constipation

- *Hydrogen sulfide:* diarrhea

Treatment

The main diet used to treat SIBO is the low-FODMAP diet. This refers to fermentable oligosaccharides, disaccharides, monosaccharides, and polyols. These are types of carbohydrates that are not well absorbed and feed the bacteria, causing fermentation and SIBO symptoms. This diet is restrictive and is not meant to be followed long-term. Generally, people follow the diet for up to four to six weeks while incorporating treatments for SIBO. A less-restrictive low-FODMAP diet can be used for a time that goes beyond four weeks, especially once you pinpoint foods that commonly aggravate your symptoms. Restricted foods include many fruits (avocados, apricots, cherries, nectarines, peaches, plums) and fructose-containing foods and drinks, dairy, wheat, garlic, onions, beans, lentils, and artificial sweeteners. Allowable foods include red meat, turkey, fish, chicken, eggs, grapes, oranges, blueberries, rice, quinoa, oats, corn, potato, many vegetables, almond milk, coconut yogurt, and teas except chamomile, chai, oolong, and fennel. There are plenty of resources available online for foods to avoid and foods to eat on the low-FODMAP diet.

Consume prebiotic and probiotic recipes in Chapter 9 that are in line with the low-FODMAP diet for the first six weeks. Once you are doing better, increase the diversity of recipes for prebiotic and probiotic foods.

Supplement with herbal formulas used for SIBO. Common ingredients include oregano, sage, thyme, berberine, bilberry, allicin, grape seed, and others. Use formulas as directed.

Supplement with the following:

- Probiotics to establish microbiome balance
- Digestive enzymes to reduce SIBO symptoms
- Psyllium seed fiber to help bowel movements
- Milk thistle for bile flow support to reduce SIBO symptoms
- Bitters or betaine hydrochloride with meals

For SIBO cases that are severe or not responsive to herbal therapy, antibiotics may be used in conjunction with diet and supplement recommendations.

ULCERS

Ulcers refer to open sores that line the stomach (peptic ulcer) or the first part of the small intestine (duodenal ulcer). The resulting symptoms can be a burning pain in the upper or mid abdomen, feeling of fullness, belching, bloating, heartburn, nausea, loss of appetite, bloody or black stool (from bleeding), and vomiting that could include blood. Ulcers can be very serious and life-threatening and therefore treatment needs to be supervised by a doctor. Conventional therapy with acid-suppressing medications along with natural therapies may be required.

The most common causes of ulcers include infection with the bacteria *H. pylori* and the use of nonsteroidal anti-inflammatory drugs (aspirin, ibuprofen, and naproxen). Up to 20 percent of people who regularly take NSAIDs develop ulcers, and 3 percent develop bowel hemorrhage or perforation. These causes eliminate the natural mucus layer of the stomach and small intestine. As a result, stomach acid damages the mucosal lining. If you have a duodenal ulcer, then leaky gut will be present.

Treatment

The holistic treatment of ulcers involves the same treatment for gastritis. In addition, patients who are anemic may require iron and B_{12} supplementation. Make sure to use more gentle forms of iron such as bisglycinate instead of forms like ferrous sulfate, which cause GI irritation.

○ ○ ◎ ○ ○

While it's not surprising that a leaky gut would be connected to digestive issues, many people don't expect it to be linked to so many other conditions like joint pain, heart disease, anxiety, eczema, or insomnia. In the next chapter we'll explore these non-digestive conditions and the holistic therapies that can help alleviate their symptoms.

Chapter 8

PROTOCOLS FOR TARGETING NON-DIGESTIVE CONDITIONS

Paul, a 40-year-old businessman, had a flare up of his IBS in recent months. In addition, he was feeling depressed and had muscle soreness from normal amounts of physical activity. His IBS symptoms were mainly related to the unhealthy diet he had been consuming. He stated that his stress level was not high. I recommended we treat his digestion first and then see what symptoms remained. After 30 days of closely following my diet recommendations and supplement regimen, he noticed his mood and muscle soreness were no longer problematic. When we followed up six months later, he continued to be symptom free.

As I discussed in Chapters 1 and 2, there is a gut relationship with all the systems of the body. In the last chapter we focused on digestive issues, but a leaky gut can cause so many other ailments. It has even been linked to post-COVID syndrome. In this chapter I will provide some additional integrative and holistic approaches that complement gut healing for successfully addressing the following conditions, in alphabetical order:

- acne

- adrenal dysfunction

- allergies and asthma

- anxiety

- autoimmunity

- bone health: osteopenia and osteoporosis

- cardiovascular health

- depression

- diabetes and prediabetes

- diabetic retinopathy

- eczema

- fatigue

- hair, nails, and skin health

- hypothyroidism

- insomnia

- joint pain and osteoarthritis

- macular degeneration

- memory and concentration

- menopause

- nervous system balance

- premenstrual syndrome (PMS)

- psoriasis

- testosterone deficiency in males

- vision issues

- weight issues: higher weight, hormone imbalances, and metabolism

- weight issues: lower weight and malabsorption

ACNE

The skin is a large organ and is generally resilient to disease. However, a number of factors can make you susceptible to skin conditions, such as injuries and infections, inflammatory conditions, cancer, and abnormal pigmenting. About one in four Americans have a skin condition. Skin conditions often arise from imbalances within the body. Researchers have noted that digestive disorders are often accompanied by skin conditions, especially when the microbiome is imbalanced.

One of the categories of internal disharmony associated with skin conditions is leaky gut and dysbiosis. *Frontiers in Microbiology* reported "an intimate, bidirectional connection between the gut and skin, and numerous studies link gastrointestinal (GI) health to skin homeostasis and allostasis."[1] Many people with chronic skin conditions notice improvement when they improve intestinal health due to the gut-skin axis.

The American Academy of Dermatology reports that acne (acne vulgaris type) affects up to 50 million Americans annually.[2] The condition is more common in adolescents and young adults but also can occur into the third and fourth decade of life. Hormonal changes can play a role in the formation of acne.

The *Journal of Clinical Medicine* reported that the gut microbiota affects the skin microbiota, and that the intestinal flora may aggravate acne.[3] The same researchers reported that probiotics directly inhibit the bacteria *Cutibacterium acnes*, a bacteria located on the skin known to be involved in acne inflammation.

See also the section in this chapter: Hair, Nails, and Skin Health on page 167.

Treatment

For some people diet has a pronounced effect on acne, while for others it has little to no effect. Chocolate, dairy products, and sugar can be aggravating food items for some. The industrialized Western diet is thought to play a role in acne (and certainly in skin inflammation). The Modified Mediterranean Diet in Chapter 9 supports healthy skin, as it is dairy and gluten free, and low in simple sugars. Additional therapies to consider include:

- *Zinc:* This mineral can help reduce acne formation.[4] Take 50 to 100 mg daily, with 2 mg of copper, with a meal.

- *Tea tree oil:* The topical use of tea tree oil products has been shown to significantly improve mild to moderate acne.[5] Use products designed for topical applications.

- *Prebiotics and probiotics:* Take/consume daily to balance the microbiome. There are now several studies demonstrating that oral and topical probiotics improve acne.[6]

- *Liver-cleansing herbs:* Combination formulas including potent ingredients such as milk thistle, dandelion root, turmeric, and artichoke are readily available. Use as directed on the label. The liver is involved in detoxification.

ADRENAL DYSFUNCTION

There is a direct communication system between the gut microbiota and hormones produced in the gut with the hormonal glands. As discussed in Chapter 2, leaky gut creates systemic inflammation, which can lead to a cascade of events that disrupts the hormonal systems. Also, dysbiosis of the microbiome negatively influences the hormones released by gut cells that affect many metabolic processes. The treatment of chronic hormone imbalances can be helped by treating leaky gut and dysbiosis. I will review some of the major hormonal conditions associated with leaky gut and dysbiosis, and additional helpful therapies for a well-rounded approach.

The two adrenal glands located on top of the kidneys are a critical component of the body's ability to adapt to stress. Adrenal hormones play major roles in the functioning of the body and are required for life. After being synthesized and released by the adrenal glands, they travel in the bloodstream and act on a variety of tissues to carry out their functions. Examples of adrenal hormones include cortisol, DHEA, pregnenolone, epinephrine, norepinephrine, and others. Testing with saliva, blood, or urine can help pinpoint hormonal imbalances.

The adrenal glands do not work in isolation. They are a component of a larger stress response system. The limbic-hypothalamic-pituitary axis (LHPA) is the main response system the body uses to cope and adapt to stress. Intense stress, illness, toxins, and various chronic stressors (mental, emotional, spiritual) can lead to an imbalance in adrenal hormones. Such imbalances can cause a host of problems that range from fatigue, a weak immune system, autoimmunity, anxiety, depression, muscle weakness, poor metabolism, cognitive problems, digestive problems, and increased risk of imbalance with other hormonal systems.

Treatment

Stress-reduction techniques (as discussed in Chapter 6) are essential to balancing the LHPA and adrenal hormones. The Modified Mediterranean Diet in Chapter 9 is a good choice to provide an environment for adrenal hormone balance.

Additional therapies to consider:

- *Ashwagandha:* Shown in several studies to improve resistance to stress,[7] it has a balancing effect on the LHPA. It also reduces cortisol and improves DHEA levels, mood, and sleep. Take 250 mg to 500 mg of a standardized extract daily.

- *Rhodiola:* An adaptogenic herb that helps the body and hormonal system adapt to stress, rhodiola has many benefits, including helping with mental fatigue.[8] Take 200 to 300 mg of a standardized product daily.

- *CBD (Cannabinoids):* Supplements derived from hemp and containing various CBDs are available without the psychoactive compound THC (tetrahydrocannabinol). The body has an endocannabinoid system with receptors for various cannabinoids. CBD can help with stress and anxiety and insomnia. In addition, it has an anti-inflammatory effect on the nervous system. Take as directed on the label.

- *Multivitamin:* A good multivitamin formula supplies the body with nutrients needed for hormone metabolism.

- *Prebiotics and probiotics:* Take/consume daily to balance the microbiome.

In more severe cases of adrenal dysfunction, an integrative doctor can prescribe bioidentical hormones, such as pregnenolone, DHEA, and cortisol.

ALLERGIES AND ASTHMA

Allergies and asthma are intertwined with one another. Over 50 million Americans experience allergies each year.[9] This occurs when the immune system reacts to a substance as if it were dangerous. This section will focus on environmental allergies. About 8 percent of U.S. adults and 7 percent of children have seasonal allergic rhinitis, also known as hay fever. Research published in *Internal Archives of Allergy and Immunology* revealed that adults with allergic rhinitis have a reduced microbiome diversity.[10] Additional research published in *Nature Reviews: Immunology* reported an association of allergic rhinitis and leaky gut.[11]

It is estimated that more than 25 million Americans have asthma.[12] With this condition the airway becomes inflamed and constricted, making it difficult to breathe. One of the triggers of asthma is allergies, such as allergic rhinitis. Other triggers include pollution, smoke, dust mites, stress, weather changes, temperature changes, fragrances and scents, and exercise. *Physiological Reviews* revealed that about 40 percent of people with asthma have leaky gut.[13] People on asthma medications should not stop or alter medication use without the guidance of a doctor.

Treatment

A diet that is rich in antioxidants and low in refined carbohydrates can benefit those with allergies and asthma. People with multiple food sensitivities likely have leaky gut and dysbiosis, and food sensitivities should be identified and treated, and problematic foods should be restricted or rotated. The Modified Mediterranean Diet in Chapter 9 supports allergies and asthma, as it is dairy and gluten free, low in simple sugars, and rich in antioxidants and inflammation-reducing fatty acids. The following supplements can also help alleviate allergies and asthma:

- *Quercetin:* This flavonoid has natural antihistamine effects. Research has shown that quercetin significantly reduces allergic rhinitis symptoms, such as eye itching, sneezing, nasal discharge, and sleep disruptions, compared to placebos.[14] In addition, quercetin has been shown to improve asthma and allergic rhinitis when combined with conventional treatment compared to conventional treatment only.[15] Take 250 mg twice daily of the phytosome type for high bioavailability.

- *Pycnogenol:* This extract from pine bark has been shown to improve mild to moderate asthma symptoms and its effects have been studied in children.[16] Take 100 mg daily or as directed by your healthcare provider.

- *N-acetylcysteine (NAC):* This compound thins
  mucus that can be problematic with allergies and
  asthma. Take 500 to 600 mg twice daily on an
  empty stomach.

- *Magnesium:* This mineral acts as a relaxer of the
  airway. Take 250 to 500 mg daily.

- *Prebiotics and probiotics:* Take/consume daily to
  balance the microbiome.

ANXIETY

Approximately 19 percent of adults in the U.S. have anxiety. There are different types of anxiety disorders, but common
themes include excessive worry or fear. There are many different
causes, ranging from psychological to genetic to physical. *Clinics
and Practice* reported that dysbiosis and inflammation of the gut
are linked to anxiety.[17]

See also the section in this chapter: Nervous System Balance
on page 177.

Treatment

For some people a focus on improving gut health may result in
improved mood, so the Modified Mediterranean Diet in Chapter
9 is a good place to start. The following supplements can also help
alleviate symptoms:

- *Gamma-aminobutyric acid (GABA):* This amino acid
  has a calming effect on the brain.[18] Take 200 mg to
  500 mg one to three times daily.

- *L-theanine:* This is another amino acid that has a
  calming effect on the brain.[19] Take 200 mg one to
  three times daily.

- *Magnesium:* Take 250 to 500 mg daily to relax the
  brain and nervous system.

- *Ashwagandha:* This adaptogen has been shown to improve resistance to stress and improve mood. Take 125 to 250 mg of an extract daily.

- *CBD (Cannabinoids):* Look for supplements derived from hemp that contain various CBDs but do not contain the psychoactive compound THC (tetrahydrocannabinol). The body has an endocannabinoid system with receptors for various cannabinoids. CBD can help with stress and anxiety.[20] Take as directed on the label.

- *Prebiotics and probiotics:* Take/consume daily to balance the microbiome.

AUTOIMMUNITY

Autoimmunity refers to a group of diseases in which the immune system mounts an attack against its own tissues. There are more than 100 known autoimmune conditions. Some of the more common autoimmune conditions include rheumatoid arthritis, Hashimoto's thyroiditis, Crohn's disease, type 1 diabetes, multiple sclerosis, psoriasis, Sjogren's syndrome, and lupus erythematosus. Symptoms common to autoimmunity include fatigue, joint swelling and pain, skin problems, digestive problems, recurring fever, and swollen glands.[21] According to conventional medicine, risk factors include genetics, being at a higher weight, smoking, and taking some medications. However, as I explained in Chapter 2, there is strong evidence that leaky gut and dysbiosis are commonly involved in the predisposition to autoimmune disease. *Nature Reviews Immunology* reported a tremendous increase in autoimmune diseases worldwide and noted that these diseases are more prevalent in industrialized countries.[22] It proposed that dysfunction and inflammation in the intestinal epithelial cells (leaky gut) and dysbiosis are causative factors with autoimmunity.

Treatment

A gluten-free diet is strongly advised for people with an auto-immune condition. I also recommend a diet that lowers inflammation through whole foods. The Modified Mediterranean Diet in Chapter 9 can provide an environment for healthy immune function. Intermittent fasting under a practitioner's supervision can also be helpful for some people with autoimmunity.

The supplements recommended for leaky gut and dysbiosis in Chapter 5 are advisable for most people with autoimmunity. Additional supplements that can help include:

- *Omega-3 fatty acids:* These reduce the inflammatory response of the immune system. Take 1000 mg to 2000 mg of EPA and DHA combined daily.

- *L-glutathione:* This antioxidant supports detoxification and reduces inflammation. Take 500 mg twice daily on an empty stomach.

- *Prebiotics and probiotics:* Take/consume daily to balance the microbiome.

In addition, consult with an integrative doctor to make sure your hormones are balanced, especially the adrenal hormones, which regulate immunity and inflammation. The medication known as LDN (low-dose naltrexone) is used by integrative doctors for several autoimmune conditions to modulate the immune system.

BONE HEALTH: OSTEOPENIA AND OSTEOPOROSIS

The gut-bone axis is recognized as playing a role in bone density. As with other conditions, osteoporosis is a disease of chronic inflammation. (Osteopenia is a loss of bone mass or bone mineral density, and it is the stage before osteoporosis.)

The presence of leaky gut and dysbiosis are major players when it comes to inflammation. Research has shown that menopausal women have increased gut permeability, which is associated with more inflammation and lower bone mineral density.[23] In a study of women ages 75 to 80 years old who had low bone mineral density and were given a probiotic or placebo, those receiving the probiotic for one year had reduced loss of bone compared to those given the placebo.[24]

Treatment

The Modified Mediterranean Diet in Chapter 9 is protective against bone loss. There is no one nutrient that supports bone building but rather a team of nutrients. Proper diet, weight-bearing exercise, and supplementation as a multifactorial approach is best in improving bone density. Bone formulas containing many of the ingredients in one formula are readily available. The following can all be helpful:

- *Vitamin D:* Take 2000 IU to 5000 IU daily with food, depending on blood level.

- *Calcium:* Take 500 mg one to two times daily with meals (depending on dietary intake).

- *Magnesium:* Take 250 to 500 mg daily.

- *Vitamin K_2:* Take 500 mcg or higher (consult with your doctor).

- *Omega-3 fatty acids:* Take 1000 mg of EPA and DHA combined.

- *Silicon:* Take 10 mg daily.

- *Resveratrol:* Take 500 mg daily.[25]

- *Probiotic:* Take a formula with human-studied strains daily.

CARDIOVASCULAR HEALTH

Cardiovascular disease refers to problems of the heart and blood vessels and may include coronary heart disease, blood clots, cerebrovascular disease (diseased blood vessels affecting the brain), peripheral arterial disease, and others. People with cardiovascular disease are also more susceptible to stroke and heart attack. High blood pressure, lipid imbalance, genetics, poor nutritional status, smoking, diabetes, and other causes are risk factors. Approximately half of all American adults will have some type of cardiovascular disease in their lifetime. There is a relationship between gut health and cardiovascular health, and the gut-heart axis is recognized for both dysbiosis and leaky gut.

Treatment

The Modified Mediterranean Diet in Chapter 9 has been shown in many studies to be protective against many types of cardiovascular disease. In addition to addressing leaky gut and dysbiosis, consider the following therapies:

- *Omega-3 fatty acids:* These reduce cardiovascular inflammation and improve blood flow. Take 1000 mg of EPA and DHA combined daily.

- *Magnesium:* This mineral supports normal heart contraction and relaxes blood vessels for improved blood flow. Take 250 to 500 mg daily.

- *Multivitamin:* These formulas can provide antioxidants, such as full-spectrum Vitamin E and others, to protect against LDL oxidation. LDL oxidation is a fundamental reason that inflammation in the blood vessels occur. Take as directed on the label.

- *Coenzyme Q10:* This antioxidant supports normal heart contraction and improves circulation. Take 100 to 200 mg daily.

- *Garlic and garlic extracts:* Supplmenting with garlic can improve lipid profiles. Garlic also has a natural anticoagulant benefit. Take as directed on the label.

- *Vitamin K_2:* This vitamin may prevent excessive calcification of the arteries. Take 100 mcg to 500 mcg daily.

- *Red yeast rice and bergamot extract:* If you have cholestorol abnormalities, daily intake of these supplements (2400 mg red yeast rice and 2000 mg bergamot extract) may be recommended by your holistic doctor.

- *Prebiotics and probiotics:* Take/consume daily to balance the microbiome.

DEPRESSION

Depression refers to ongoing symptoms of sadness and often a loss of interest in daily activities. The severity of depression can range from mild to severe. There are several other symptoms that can occur, such as insomnia, fatigue, changes in appetite, poor concentration, thoughts of suicide or death, and more. This condition is diagnosed by a healthcare professional based on your signs and symptoms. It is estimated that between 6 and 7 percent of U.S. adults have depression.

The causes of depression can be situational and/or biochemical, but dysbiosis and inflammation of the gut are also linked to depression.[26]

See also the section in this chapter: Nervous System Balance on page 177.

Treatment

The Modified Mediterranean Diet in Chapter 9 can provide an environment in the body conducive to nervous system balance.

Make sure to get adequate omega-3 fatty acids for nervous system health. The following supplements can also help alleviate the symptoms of depression:

- *5-hydroxytryptophan (5-HTP):* This amino acid supports production of the neurotransmitter serotonin. Take 100 mg three times daily on an empty stomach.

- *Saffron:* The extract from this spice has been shown to support mood and improve symptoms of depression.[27]

- *Ashwagandha:* This adaptogen has been shown to improve mood and resistance to stress. Take 125 to 250 mg of an extract daily.

- *Omega-3 fatty acids:* These support brain neurotransmitter production and reduce inflammation of the brain. Take 1000 mg of EPA and DHA combined daily.

- *Prebiotics and probiotics:* Take/consume daily to balance the microbiome.

DIABETES AND PREDIABETES

Elevated glucose and insulin levels in children and adults is problematic in the United States and around the world. Poor diet and being at a higher weight are the main causes of prediabetes and type 2 diabetes. However, as discussed in Chapter 2, people with diabetes are more likely to have leaky gut and dysbiosis. The imbalanced microbiota of the gut contributes to insulin resistance.

Treatment

In addition to addressing leaky gut and dysbiosis, a reduced carbohydrate diet can help, especially one that is low in simple carbohydrates, combined with high fiber, moderate protein, and moderate good fat. The Modified Mediterranean Diet is a good choice for many people with diabetes and prediabetes. More restrictive diets may be followed under the guidance of a knowledgeable practitioner. In addition, intermittent fasting is effective in reducing and managing glucose levels.

You may also want to consider the following additional therapies:

- *Berberine:* An extract from Indian barberry, it has been shown in several studies to be effective in reducing glucose levels for those with Type 2 diabetes and insulin resistance.[28] A typical dose is 500 mg two to three times daily.

- *Soluble fiber:* Taken before meals, a soluble fiber formula reduces glucose absorption in the gut and prevents insulin spiking. Take as directed on the container.

- *Multivitamin and mineral formula:* Take daily to address the many nutrients involved in glucose metabolism.

- *Turmeric extract:* Tumeric has been shown to lower glucose levels. Look for a product that supplies 300 mg per day of curcuminoids.

- *Prebiotics and probiotics:* Take/consume daily to balance the microbiome.

Regular exercise is critical for those with prediabetes and diabetes to manage glucose levels. Consider continuous glucose monitoring systems to evaluate how your diet and program is working.

DIABETIC RETINOPATHY

This condition occurs in people with diabetes and is caused by damage to blood vessels in the retina. About one-third of adults over the age of 40 in the U.S. have diabetic retinopathy. In the later stages of the disease, you may see floaters such as spots or streaks. This condition can also cause diabetic macular edema, neovascular glaucoma, and retinal detachment.

See also the sections in this chapter: Diabetes and Prediabetes on page 162 and Vision Issues on page 182.

Treatment

The best way to prevent and treat this condition is through glucose management. Proper diet, exercise, weight balance, stress reduction, supplements, and, if needed, medications can help. Follow the same recommendations for macular degeneration, along with the following supplement:

- *Pycnogenol:* This compound improves circulation to the retina and reduces tissue swelling.[29] Take 100 to 150 mg daily.

ECZEMA

Eczema, also known as atopic dermatitis, is characterized by dry and itchy skin. There are different types of eczema, and it can affect people of all ages. Up to 25 percent of children and 10 percent of adults in the United States have some degree of eczema.[30] There are several known causes of eczema, including genetics, climate (often worse in cold and damp climates), stress, pollution, and tobacco smoke. Additional causes addressed by holistic doctors include environmental allergens, diet, nutritional deficiencies, and gut health. Food sensitivities play a definite role for many people with eczema. Essential fatty acids, especially omega-3s, are often low or deficient in those with eczema. Essential fatty acids not only reduce skin inflammation but also play a role in maintaining moisture.

The health and development of the microbiome and risk of allergy is influenced early in life (during the prenatal period and first two years of life) through factors such as natural birth, breast-feeding, contact with nature and pets, appropriate diet, and the consumption of prebiotics and probiotics.[31] Leaky gut is associated with food allergies, and food allergies are known triggers of eczema.[32]

See also the section in this chapter: Hair, Nails, and Skin Health on page 167.

Treatment

The Modified Mediterranean Diet in Chapter 9 supports healthy skin, as it is dairy and gluten free, and low in simple sugars. The following supplements can also help alleviate eczema:

- *Omega-3 fatty acids:* Omega-3s reduce skin inflammation and help maintain skin hydration. Adults should take 1000 mg of EPA and DHA combined twice daily. Children should take a quarter to half that amount as directed by their healthcare provider. It should be noted that some people with eczema also benefit from gamma-linoleic acid (GLA) in addition to omega-3 supplementation.

- *Multivitamin:* A good multivitamin formula supplies several of the vitamins and minerals involved in skin health.

- *Vitamin D:* This vitamin plays a role in controlling skin inflammation. Have your blood levels tested and supplement with 2000 IU to 5000 IU daily if you're low.

- *Prebiotics and probiotics:* Take/consume daily to balance the microbiome. Studies show that one should take probiotics for at least eight weeks before assessing efficacy.[33]

FATIGUE

Fatigue is common among adults and is characterized by the reduced capacity for physical and/or mental activity. There are many reasons for fatigue, including stress, insomnia, hormone and neurotransmitter imbalances, chronic illnesses and infections, nutrient deficiencies (iron, B_{12}, B_1, CoQ10), side effects of medications, and others.

Improving gut and microbiome health can be effective in helping those with long-term fatigue. One of the obvious reasons improved gut health can improve energy levels is that it optimizes the absorption of nutrients. Cellular energy production requires a host of nutrients in producing the body's energy currency known as adenosine triphosphate (ATP). And as I discussed in Chapter 2, the metabolites of microbiota activity produce short-chain fatty acids that stimulate energy production in the cell energy factories known as mitochondria. When you have dysbiosis and malabsorption, it creates a toxic load that not only diverts energy for detoxification but also interferes with cellular energy production. Then there is the issue of inflammation with poor gut health. Inflammation interferes with mitochondrial energy production. Also, chronic infections in the gut create inflammation and can damage intestinal health. And last, poor gut health and digestion disrupts glucose metabolism, which ultimately makes energy production less efficient.

Treatment

The Modified Mediterranean Diet in Chapter 9 supports cellular energy production. It is low in simple carbohydrates and has energy-sustaining fatty acids as well as antioxidants for mitochondrial health. The following supplements can also help with fatigue:

- *B complex:* These vitamins are important for cellular energy production. Take daily as directed on the label.

- *Coenzyme Q10 (ubiquinone, ubiquinol):* This antioxident supports energy production in the cell. Take 200 mg to 400 mg daily.

- *Ashwagandha:* This adaptogen has been shown to increase resistance to stress and increase energy levels. Take 125 to 250 mg of an extract daily.

- *Nicotinamide adenine dinucleotide NAD+:* This supports cellular energy production. Take 500 mg daily.

- *D-ribose:* This naturally occurring sugar is available as a supplement that supports cell energy. Take 5 grams two to three times daily.

- *Acetyl-L-carnitine:* This amino acid helps fat to be burned as fuel. Take 1000 mg twice daily between meals.

- *Prebiotics and probiotics:* Take/consume daily to balance the microbiome.

HAIR, NAILS, AND SKIN HEALTH

While the hair, nails, and skin are outer coverings of the body, they often reflect the inner activities of the gut. Chronic problems like hair loss, dry skin, and brittle nails are often related at least in part to leaky gut and dysbiosis.

See also the sections in this chapter: Acne on page 151, Eczema on page 164, and Psoriasis on page 179.

Treatment

Additional natural therapies for brittle hair and nails and hair loss include:

- *Silica:* This form of silicon can improve hair growth and quality and address brittle nails. Take 10 mg daily of choline-stabilized orthosilicic acid.

- *Biotin:* This B vitamin supports healthy hair and nail growth. Take 2000 mcg to 5000 mcg daily. Topical solutions such as shampoos that contain biotin can also be used daily.

- *Multivitamin and mineral formula:* Take daily to address other nutritional deficiencies that could be related to hair and/or nail problems.

- *Omega-3 fatty acids:* Omega-3s are required for healthy hair and nails. Take 1000 mg of EPA and DHA combined daily.

- *Methylsulfonylmethane (MSM):* This compound has been shown to support hair and nail growth. Take 3000 mg daily.

- *Betaine hydrochloride and pepsin:* These enzymes mimic stomach acid to improve nutrient absorption. Take one to two capsules with a meal (reduce the dose or stop if you have a warm or burning sensation in the gut). Another option is to take a bitters herbal formula before meals.

Also have your iron and iron stores (ferritin) checked by your doctor. If they're low, iron supplementation can help hair growth and abnormal nail shape and poor growth. Talk to a specialist about the use of an FDA-approved laser cap used to stimulate hair growth. Or talk to a doctor who uses platelet-rich plasma (PRP) to stimulate hair growth.

Additional natural therapies for skin include:

- *Collagen peptides:* Collagen supports healthy skin and for some forms, human studies have shown that taking collagen peptides improves skin wrinkling.

- *Silica:* This form of silicon can improve skin health and possibly reduce wrinkles. Take 10 mg daily of choline-stabilized orthosilicic acid.

- *Multivitamin and mineral formula:* Take daily to address other nutritional deficiencies that could be related to skin problems.

- *Omega-3 fatty acids:* Omega-3s are required for skin health, especially for dry skin. Take 1000 mg of EPA and DHA combined daily.

- *Betaine hydrochloride and pepsin:* These enzymes mimic stomach acid to improve nutrient absorption. Take one to two capsules with a meal (reduce the dose or stop if you have a warm or burning sensation in the gut). Another option is to take a bitters herbal formula before meals.

Also consider that the skin reflects the detoxification processes of the inner body. Chronic skin conditions may be helped by supporting liver and kidney detoxification. Formulas that contain herbs such as milk thistle and other gentle detox supportive agents can be helpful. You should be aware that food sensitivities can lead to skin rashes, eczema, and psoriasis flare-ups in some people.

HYPOTHYROIDISM

Hypothyroidism or low thyroid is a very common condition. Low levels of thyroid hormones can cause fatigue, weight gain, cold intolerance, loss of hair and eyebrows, depression, constipation, and several other symptoms.

The most common cause by far for hypothyroidism is an autoimmune condition known as Hashimoto's thyroiditis (HT). HT is an autoimmune disease in which the immune system attacks thyroid gland tissue and makes you susceptible to the underproduction of thyroid hormones.

As reported in *Frontiers in Immunology*, "There is a lot of evidence that the intestinal dysbiosis, bacterial overgrowth, and increased intestinal permeability (leaky gut) favor HT development, and a thyroid-gut axis has been proposed which seems to impact our entire metabolism."[34]

See also the section in this chapter: Autoimmunity on page 157.

Treatment

The Modified Mediterranean Diet in Chapter 9 provides an environment for adrenal hormone balance. If you consume a lot of cruciferous vegetables (e.g., broccoli, cauliflower, cabbage, kale, bok choy, arugula, and Brussel sprouts), make sure they are cooked or steamed to reduce goitrogens that may inhibit iodine uptake by the thyroid. The following supplements can also help balance your adrenal hormones:

- *Myo-inositol combined with selenium:* A formulation of 600 mg myo-inositol plus 83 mcg selenium has been shown in several studies to reduce thyroid antibodies and improve thyroid hormone levels.[35]

- *Multivitamin:* A good mulivitamin supplies the nutrients needed for hormone metabolism. Make sure to have a daily intake of 100 to 200 mcg of selenium as part of your multivitamin.

- *Prebiotics and probiotics:* Take/consume daily to balance the microbiome.

Do not supplement iodine at higher doses (more than 200 mcg), unless a practitioner evaluates your iodine status before supplementation and monitors your condition.

INSOMNIA

Difficulty falling or staying asleep are the hallmarks of insomnia. This condition occurs in about 30 percent of adults in the United States.[36] There are several known causes of insomnia, such as diet (alcohol); stress; nutrient deficiencies (B_{12}, iron); medical conditions such as apnea, restless leg syndrome, and others; and hormonal imbalances.

There is emerging evidence regarding the gut-brain-microbiota axis and how it affects sleep. It is now known that the microbiota influences circadian rhythms, such as the sleep cycle. *Frontiers in Psychiatry* reported evidence that gut microbiota interacts with genes that modulate the sleep cycle.[37] Researchers have found that certain gut microbiota were correlated negatively with sleep measures.[38]

Treatment

For some people a healthy diet causes a big improvement in their insomnia. The Modified Mediterranean Diet in Chapter 9 can support proper biochemistry for sleep. Make sure to avoid caffeine, alcohol, and sugar in the evening, and try not to eat late at night. I also recommend steering clear of light sources at bedtime, including phones, television, and computer screens. Regular exercise is effective in alleviating insomnia. The following supplements can also help with insomnia:

- *Melatonin:* This is a natural hormone that induces the sleep cycle. Take 1 to 5 mg one hour before bedtime. If you can fall asleep but wake up, then use the time-released form (3 to 5 mg).

- *L-theanine:* This amino acid is calming to the brain and can help normalize the sleep cycle. Take 200 to 500 mg a half hour before bedtime.

- *Passionflower root:* This plant can calm the brain and nervous system. Take 300 to 500 mg of the capsule form a half hour before bedtime.

- *Ashwagandha:* This adaptogen has been shown to reduce the effects of stress and improve sleep. Take 125 to 250 mg of an extract daily.

- *CBD (Cannabinoids):* Look for supplements derived from hemp that contain various CBDs but do not contain the psychoactive compound THC (tetrahydrocannabinol). The body has an endocannabinoid system with receptors for various cannabinoids. CBD can help with stress and anxiety that may be triggering insomnia. Take as directed on the label a half hour before bedtime.

- *Prebiotics and probiotics:* Take/consume daily to balance the microbiome.

JOINT PAIN AND OSTEOARTHRITIS

Osteoarthritis is the most common form of arthritis that occurs from joint cartilage breakdown. Approximately 32.5 million U.S. adults have osteoarthritis.[39] The gut-joint axis is real and discussed in Chapter 2. Essentially, leaky gut and dysbiosis create an environment of inflammation that affects the joints. Improvements in gut health reduce systemic inflammation that worsens osteoarthritis.

See also the section in this chapter: Autoimmunity on page 157 (for autoimmune arthritis).

Treatment

The Modified Mediterranean Diet in Chapter 9 works well to reduce body and joint inflammation. In addition to addressing leaky gut and dysbiosis, consider the following therapies:

- *Omega-3 fatty acids:* Omega-3s are required for joint health and to reduce joint inflammation and stiffness. Take 1000 mg of EPA and DHA combined daily.

- *Glucosamine sulfate:* This amino sugar supports cartilage and reduces pain and stiffness.[40] Take 1500 mg daily.

- *Type II collagen:* Use a form that has been studied for the treatment of osteoarthritis.[41] Available in capsule or powder form.

- *Methylsulfonylmethane (MSM):* This compound reduces inflammation and provides sulfur for cartilage formation. Take 3000 to 5000 mg daily.

- *Turmeric extract:* This spice reduces inflammation and stiffness. Take 500 mg two to three times daily.

- *Prebiotics and probiotics:* Take/consume daily to balance the microbiome.

Additional holistic therapies include acupuncture, physical therapy, and regenerative injection therapies, such as those involving ozone injections, platelet-rich plasma, and stem cells.

MACULAR DEGENERATION

There are two main types of macular degeneration with different pathologies: atrophic or dry and neovascular or wet. The macula is the portion of the retina that manages sharp, central vision. I will focus on atrophic macular degeneration, also referred to as age-related macular degeneration.

See also the section in this chapter: Vision Issues on page 182.

Treatment

I recommend a diet rich in antioxidants, especially carotenoids. Lutein and zeaxanthin are the most-studied carotenoids to date for macular degeneration. Foods rich in these carotenoids include kale, collards, spinach, broccoli, green peas, turnip greens, eggs, carrots, and oranges. The following carotenoids are important for macular health:

- *Lutein:* Take 10 to 15 mg daily with food.

- *Zeaxanthin:* Take 3 mg daily with a meal.

- *Astaxanthin:* Take 1000 to 3000 mcg daily.

Omega-3 fatty acids are also important to reduce inflammation. The Modified Mediterranean Diet in Chapter 9 supports retina and macula health. Research in *Ophthalmology* reported that the Mediterranean diet is associated with a 41 percent reduced risk of incidence of age-related macular degeneration.[42] Additional supplements that can help include:

- *Zinc:* This mineral acts as an antioxidant to reduce macular degeneration. Take 25 to 50 mg daily with a meal.

- *Bilberry:* This berry contains flavonoids that nourish the retina. Take 300 to 600 mg daily of an extract.

- *Fish oil:* Consuming fish oil supplies omega-3 fatty acids, which reduce inflammation. Take 1000 mg of EPA and DHA combined daily.

- *Prebiotics and probiotics:* Take/consume daily to balance the microbiome.

MEMORY AND CONCENTRATION

The ability to store and retrieve memories can be a challenge for people of many different ages, but as we grow older, we are more susceptible to age-related memory impairment and even dementia. There are many factors that can contribute to poor memory and concentration. These include stress, certain illnesses, nutrient deficiencies, hormone imbalances, neurotransmitter imbalance, genetics, and other factors. The gut-brain-microbiota axis influences learning and cognitive function.[43] A study in the journal *Brain, Behavior, & Immunity—Health* reported an association between leaky gut and dysbiosis with cognitive decline.[44]

See also the section in this chapter: Nervous System Balance on page 177.

Treatment

Being physically and mentally active are important in preventing memory and concentration problems. Proper nutrition is also essential for healthy brain functioning. The Modified Mediterranean Diet in Chapter 9 can provide an environment for brain health. Make sure to get adequate omega-3 fatty acids for optimal memory and concentration abilities. The following supplements can also help memory and concentration:

- *Citicoline:* This is a natural substance used by the brain to make the neurotransmitter acetylcholine. Studies show it supports memory.[45] Take 250 to 500 mg daily.

- *Acetyl-L-carnitine:* This amino acid supports memory through neurotransmitter production. Take 500 mg three times daily.

- *Bacopa monnieri*: This plant has been shown in research to improve cognitive function. Take 200 to 300 mg daily.[46]

- *B vitamins:* Several of the B vitamins are important for memory, especially B_{12}, folate, and B_6. Take a B complex daily. Methylated forms are generally best. If you have absorption problems, then sublingual forms can be used.

- *Omega-3 fatty acids:* Omega-3s support brain neurotransmitter production and reduce inflammation of the brain. Take 1000 mg of EPA and DHA combined daily.

- *Prebiotics and probiotics:* Take/consume daily to balance the microbiome.

MENOPAUSE

Menopause refers to the cessation of the menstrual cycle for 12 consecutive months. In the time preceding menopause and during menopause there are changes in the levels of several hormones. Approximately 75 percent of menopausal women in the United States experience hot flashes for some time. Many other symptoms can accompany the menopausal transition that vary in severity depending on the woman, such as night sweats, depression, anxiety, heart palpitations, fatigue, joint pain, skin and hair changes, and several others.

Gut permeability increases during the menopause transition, which contributes to inflammation and lower bone mineral density.[47] As I discussed in Chapter 2, the microbiome also influences hormone metabolism.

Treatment

The Modified Mediterranean Diet in Chapter 9 provides an environment for the menopausal transition, including supporting the cardiovascular system, which is more susceptible to problems during this time. The following supplements may also be helpful:

- *Black cohosh:* Taking 80 mg or more of this extract daily has been shown to reduce several menopausal symptoms.[48]

- *Maca:* Taking 500 mg twice daily of an extract can reduce menopausal symptoms.[49]

- *Rhubarb (*Rheum rhaponticum L. *root):* Taking 4 mg daily of an extract has shown to reduce several menopausal symptoms.[50]

- *Multivitamin:* A good mulivitamin formula supplies the nutrients needed for hormone metabolism. Make sure to have a daily intake of 100 to 200 mcg of selenium.

- *A bone-health-supportive formula with calcium, magnesium, and Vitamin D:* Taking this daily as directed on the label will support bone health during the menopausal transition.

- *Prebiotics and probiotics:* Take/consume daily to balance the microbiome.

In addition, bioidentical hormone replacement (of estrogen, progesterone, testosterone, and others) is available through trained doctors to help alleviate more severe menopausal symptoms. Modern research, as discussed by the North American Menopause Society, has shown hormone therapies to have a good safety rating when given in the correct dose and combination.[51]

NERVOUS SYSTEM BALANCE

One of the most well-studied gut-organ relationships is the gut-brain axis. This refers to the two-way communication between the gut (which includes the microbiome) and brain. Nerve and neurohormone messaging from the brain travel to the gut and microbiome, and neurohormone messaging originates from the microbiome and intestinal cells and travels to the brain. You can improve brain and nervous system health, and better manage anxiety, depression, irritability, and other symptoms through gut and microbiome restoration.

See also the sections in this chapter: Anxiety on page 156, Depression on page 161, and Memory and Concentration on page 174.

Treatment

Stress-reduction techniques (as discussed in Chapter 6) are essential to balancing the nervous system and improving neurological and emotional health. The Modified Mediterranean Diet in Chapter 9 provides an environment for nervous system balance. Make sure to get adequate omega-3 fatty acids for nervous system health.

PREMENSTRUAL SYNDROME (PMS)

PMS is a disorder that affects approximately 75 percent of menstruating women. Symptoms usually begin one to two weeks before menstrual flow and can include mood changes, water retention, headaches, food cravings, fatigue, poor concentration, pelvic discomfort, and various others. The gut microbiome plays a role in hormone metabolism, and research has reported an association between gut microbiota balance and premenstrual symptoms.[52]

Treatment

A diet rich in plant foods and fiber is important for hormone balance, and healthy fatty acids and a low sugar intake have been shown to reduce symptoms. The Modified Mediterranean Diet in Chapter 9 can help alleviate PMS problems. Restrict the intake of non-organic foods laden with pesticides, which are endocrine disrupters, and the use of makeup with parabens, which are hormone disruptors. The following supplements may also help to relieve PMS symptoms:

- *Vitex (chasteberry):* Take 180 to 240 mg of an extract daily for 4 to 6 months. Research shows it has a hormone-balancing effect and reduces PMS symptoms.[53]

- *Magnesium:* Take 250 mg one to two times daily. Magnesium is involved in estrogen metabolism and calms the nervous system and reduces PMS symptoms.[54]

- *B complex:* Look for a formula that contains B_6, which is shown to help hormone metabolism and reduce PMS symptoms.[55]

- *Calcium:* Take 500 mg two times daily to reduce PMS symptoms.[56]

- *Prebiotics and probiotics:* Take/consume daily to balance the microbiome.

Consider a one-to-two month protocol of liver-cleansing herbs, such as dandelion root, burdock root, and milk thistle. Liver herbal formulas are readily available and improve the liver's metabolism of hormones. For more severe cases of PMS, a holistic doctor can prescribe bioidentical progesterone therapy.

PSORIASIS

Psoriasis is an autoimmune skin condition that often causes thick, silvery, scaly patches to appear on the skin. These plaque-like lesions can become itchy and painful. The lesions can occur anywhere but are most common on the knees, elbows, lower back, and scalp. With this condition, the skin cells multiply and shed faster than normal. Psoriasis is also associated with arthritis. Approximately 2 percent of U.S. adults have psoriasis.

There is a genetic susceptibility to developing psoriasis. Triggers can include stress, skin injury, infection, cold and dry weather, tobacco, alcohol, and some medications. Additional triggers that holistic doctors investigate include hormone imbalance, food sensitivities, and poor gut health.[57] There have been many published studies on the connection between leaky gut, dysbiosis, and psoriasis. This makes sense since most of the immune system activity originates from the gut. The *International Journal of Molecular Sciences* reported that altered gut microbiota is very common in people with psoriasis.[58] The same article noted that research demonstrated that probiotics were of benefit to most psoriatic patients. *Clinics in Dermatology* even stated that, "Psoriasis is a disease characterized by leaky gut" and that "there is a decrease in bacterial diversity and overgrowth of bacteria in the small bowel."[59] It also reported that bacterial toxins (endotoxins) absorbed from the gut into the bloodstream result in toxic effects on the liver and skin.

See also the section in this chapter: Hair, Nails, and Skin Health on page 167.

Treatment

The Modified Mediterranean Diet in Chapter 9 supports healthy skin, as it is dairy and gluten free and low in simple sugars. Gluten allergy and sensitivity is quite common in people with psoriasis. The following supplements may also improve psoriasis:

- *Vitamin D:* Studies show that levels of this vitamin are significantly lower in people with psoriasis.[60] Take 5000 IU daily with a meal or as directed by a practitioner.

- *Quercetin:* This flavonoid reduces inflammation. Take 500 mg daily; the phytosome form is preferred.

- *Turmeric extract:* This spice reduces skin inflammation and supports liver function. Take 500 mg twice daily before meals. Use a highly absorbable form. Topical forms of turmeric are also available to help with psoriatic skin lesions.

- *Milk thistle:* This plant improves liver detoxification. Take 150 to 250 mg with each meal.

- *Bile acids:* Take 500 mg with each meal to help eliminate toxins associated with psoriasis.

- *Digestive enzymes:* Take with meals to reduce food reactivity and reduced inflammation.

- *Prebiotics and probiotics:* Take daily to balance the microbiome.

TESTOSTERONE DEFICIENCY IN MALES

Low testosterone is known to occur in about 40 percent of men aged 45 and older. Common symptoms of low or deficient testosterone include fatigue, loss of muscle mass, depression, low libido, erectile dysfunction, increased abdominal fat, poor memory and focus, and more. (Women can also experience testosterone deficiency, but causes, symptoms, and treatment are different.)

There are many causes of testosterone deficiency. I review these in detail in my book *Healing the Prostate: The Best Holistic Methods to Treat the Prostate and Other Common Male-Related Conditions.* Your doctor can assess your testosterone level with lab testing.

Better gut microbiome diversity is associated with higher blood testosterone levels in men.[61] The high intake of carbohydrates (including alcohol) and insulin resistance is associated with lower testosterone levels.

Treatment

The Modified Mediterranean Diet in Chapter 9 can support hormone balance and help with a testosterone deficiency. In addition, adequate sleep and exercise help create testosterone balance. The following supplements may also be beneficial:

- *Ashwagandha:* Extracts of this herb have been shown to increase blood testosterone levels significantly in men.[62] Take 600 to 675 mg daily of a standardized extract.

- *Eurycoma longifolia (Tongkat ali):* This plant has shown to stimulate the synthesis of testosterone.[63] Take 200 to 400 mg daily of an extract.

- *Multivitamin:* Take this to supply basic nutrients for testosterone production.

- *Zinc:* Men with zinc deficiency may have improved testosterone levels with supplementation. Take 25 to 50 mg daily with a meal.

- *Vitamin D:* Deficiency of this vitamin is associated with low testosterone. Take 2000 to 5000 IU daily, depending on your blood level.

- *Magnesium:* This mineral is involved in the synthesis of testosterone. Take 250 to 500 mg daily.

- *Prebiotics and probiotics:* Take/consume daily to
  balance the microbiome.

For men with severe testosterone deficiency, there are medications that can increase the testicles' production of testosterone (e.g., Clomiphene and hCG). Bioidentical testosterone therapy is also available from a doctor.

VISION ISSUES

As by now you may expect, there is a gut-eye axis. An article in *Frontiers in Microbiology* reported that changes in the gut microbiota and its metabolites cause inflammation that can lead to eye diseases.[64] It also stated that gut microbiome abnormalities are linked to eye diseases, such as uveitis, age-related macular degeneration, Sjogren's syndrome (dry eye), diabetic retinopathy, glaucoma, and infectious keratitis.

See also the sections in this chapter: Diabetic Retinopathy on page 163 and Macular Degeneration on page 173.

Treatment

More research is needed on specific probiotics used for the treatment of eye diseases. However, a randomized, double-blind, placebo-controlled human study published in *Nutrients* found the probiotic *L. paracasei* KW3110 suppressed blue-light damage to the retinal cells.[65] Participants had subjective and objective improvements for eye disorders and eye fatigue.

WEIGHT ISSUES: HIGHER WEIGHT, HORMONE IMBALANCES, AND METABOLISM

There is emerging evidence that the microbiome affects metabolism and appetite. For those who are higher than their preferred or ideal weight, it is important to establish a healthy microbiome.

There are many issues that may need to be addressed besides calorie intake, including hormone balance and one's metabolism.

Treatment

In addition to addressing leaky gut and dysbiosis, consider the following therapies, which can be effective for weight balance:

- Intermittent fasting
- Regular exercise, including interval training
- *Soluble fiber:* Taken before meals, these supplements can help reduce appetite.
- *Prebiotics and probiotics:* Take/consume daily to balance the microbiome and promote proper metabolism.

In addition, you should address potential hormone imbalances with a holistic doctor who can assess thyroid function, adrenal function, insulin resistance, and other imbalances.

WEIGHT ISSUES: LOWER WEIGHT AND MALABSORPTION

Being lower than one's ideal weight requires focused therapy to address the underlying causes. One of the causes can be malabsorption and leaky gut, which can be helped with the recommendations in this book.

Treatment

In addition to addressing leaky gut and dysbiosis consider the following therapies:

- *Digestive enzymes:* Take with meals to improve absorption.

- *Betaine hydrochloride and pepsin:* These enzymes mimic stomach acid to improve nutrient absorption. Take one to two capsules with a meal (reduce the dose or stop if you have a warm or burning sensation in the gut). Another option is to take a bitters herbal formula before meals.

- *Protein powders:* Take one with 25 grams to 50 grams of protein daily with amino acid formulas to support muscle mass.

- *Prebiotics and probiotics:* Take/consume daily to balance the microbiome and promote proper metabolism.

In addition, you should address potential hormone imbalances with a holistic doctor who can assess thyroid function, adrenal function, growth hormone, insulin resistance, and other imbalances.

o o ⊚ o o

The treatment of leaky gut and dysbiosis will go a long way in helping most common conditions. As you have seen in this chapter, there are additional integrative and holistic methods to create whole-body healing.

Chapter 9

RECIPES TO HEAL LEAKY GUT AND BALANCE YOUR MICROBIOME

As you have read throughout the book, the foods you eat can contribute to either gut health or gut disease. I have created the following recipes to help my patients and readers heal leaky gut and balance their microbiome. A diet that promotes gut health is essential for not only digestive wellness but whole body health.

There are three components to the recommended recipes. The first component is my Modified Mediterranean Diet, which is full of plant foods that reduce inflammation and create a healthy microbiome. The recipes are restricted in dairy and gluten since so many people have digestive irritation from these foods. I have included enough Modified Mediterranean recipes for you to mix and match as desired for two weeks.

The second component of this chapter is prebiotic recipes. The recipes for these foods include the type of plant-based foods that will feed the healthy microbes in your gut. The goal is to constantly nourish the friendly flora in your gut on a regular basis. These recipes can be used as snacks or as meals.

The third component includes probiotic recipes. These recipes include food sources of the friendly flora that the gut so desperately needs to function properly. These direct food sources of probiotics are the naturally occurring good bacteria that create gut and whole body health. These recipes can be used as snacks or as meals.

MODIFIED MEDITERRANEAN DIET

High-Fat Green Smoothie

1 serving • 5 minutes

Ingredients

1 cup cold water

2 tablespoons lemon juice

1 cup baby spinach

½ avocado, frozen

¼ cup fresh mint leaves, roughly chopped

1 teaspoon fresh ginger, peeled and roughly chopped

Directions

Combine all ingredients in a blender and blend until smooth. Pour into a glass.

Notes

- *Storage (for leftovers or meal prep):* Refrigerate in an airtight container for up to one day.
- *Increase sweetness:* Add frozen banana, pineapple, or apple.
- *Increase protein:* Add protein powder or collagen powder.
- *Substitute ingredient:* Use cilantro or basil instead of mint.

○ ○ ◉ ○ ○

Green Smoothie Bowl

2 servings • 10 minutes

Ingredients

2 bananas, frozen, chopped

4 cups baby spinach

1½ cups cold water

2 ice cubes

2 kiwis, peeled and chopped

2 tablespoons unsweetened coconut flakes

2 tablespoons slivered almonds

2 tablespoons hemp seeds

Directions

Add the frozen bananas, baby spinach, water, and ice cubes to a blender. Blend until smooth.

Divide between two bowls and top with rest of ingredients. Enjoy immediately.

o o ◉ o o

Chia Oats with Kiwi

4 servings • 25 minutes

Ingredients

2 cups water
2 cups rolled oats

¼ cup chia seeds
2 kiwis, peeled and chopped

Directions

In a small saucepan, bring the water to a boil, and add in the oats and chia seeds. Cook for 10 to 15 minutes or until oats are cooked through.

Divide the oatmeal between bowls and top with chia and kiwi.

Notes

- *Storage (for leftovers or meal prep):* Refrigerate in an airtight container for up to 4 days. Store the toppings separately, if possible.
- *Suggested additional toppings:* Add nuts, seeds, berries, cinnamon to taste, and/or maple syrup.

o o ◉ o o

Blueberry Overnight Oats

2 servings • 8 hours

Ingredients

¾ cup rolled oats
¾ cup unsweetened almond milk
¼ cup water
1 tablespoon chia seeds

1 tablespoon maple syrup
½ teaspoon cinnamon
½ cup blueberries
½ cup slivered almonds

Directions

Combine all ingredients except blueberries and almonds in a large container. Stir well, cover, and place in the fridge overnight (or for at least 8 hours).

Remove the oats from the fridge. Use single-serving mason jars and place a large spoonful of the oat mix in the bottom of each. Then add a layer of blueberries followed by a layer of slivered almonds. Repeat layers until all ingredients are used up.

Enjoy immediately or save for later. They may be eaten hot or cold.

Notes

- *Storage (for leftovers or meal prep):* Store the jars in the fridge until you are ready to eat. They can be kept refrigerated in an airtight container for up to 4 days.
- *Substitute ingredient:* Use another nondairy milk of your choice.

○ ○ ◉ ○ ○

Roasted Breakfast Turnips

2 servings • 30 minutes

Ingredients

1 turnip, peeled and cut in half
1 tablespoon avocado oil
¼ teaspoon paprika
¼ teaspoon cumin

¼ teaspoon sea salt
2 eggs
1 tablespoon dried chives

Directions

Preheat the oven to 350°F (177°C).

Place the halved turnips on a baking sheet and drizzle them with avocado oil. Toss the turnips with the paprika, cumin, and salt until they are evenly coated. Bake for 20 minutes or until golden and tender.

Remove the turnips from the oven and set the oven to broil. Create pockets in the turnips with a spoon or knife, and gently crack an egg into each one. Return them to the oven and broil for 4 to 5 minutes, or until the whites are set and the yolk is cooked to your liking.

Divide onto plates, garnish with dried chives!

Notes

- *Storage (for leftovers or meal prep):* Eggs are best enjoyed the same day. Turnips can be refrigerated in an airtight container for up to 2 days.
- *Add flavor:* Add chili powder or chili flakes with the other spices.
- *Suggested additional toppings:* Top with roasted peppers, guacamole, or salsa.
- *Make it vegan:* Roast the turnips with diced vegetables instead of topping them with eggs. (This is a great way to use up leftover veggies.)

○ ○ ◎ ○ ○

Black Beans, Sweet Potato, and Egg Scramble

2 servings • 35 minutes

Ingredients

2 medium sweet potatoes, cubed

1 teaspoon avocado oil

¼ teaspoon sea salt, divided

4 eggs

1½ cups cooked black beans

1 avocado, sliced

Directions

Preheat the oven to 400°F (204°C) and line a baking sheet with parchment paper. Toss the sweet potatoes with avocado oil and half the sea salt. Bake for 25 to 30 minutes or until cooked through.

Meanwhile, heat a nonstick skillet over medium heat. Crack the eggs into a bowl and season them with the remaining sea salt. Beat the eggs gently with a fork until well combined. Add the eggs to the pan and scramble them until they are cooked through.

Divide the sweet potato, scrambled eggs, and black beans evenly. Add the sliced avocado just before serving.

Notes

- *Storage (for leftovers or meal prep):* Refrigerate in an airtight container for up to 3 days. Cut up the avocado just before serving.
- *Make it vegan:* Omit the eggs, or use a tofu scramble.
- *Substitute ingredient:* Use extra virgin olive oil or coconut oil instead of avocado oil.

o o ⊙ o o

Mashed Potato and Carrot Breakfast Bowl

2 servings • 30 minutes

Ingredients

4 cups water, divided

2 russet potatoes, peeled and chopped

1 carrot, peeled and chopped

2 eggs, hard boiled

2 tablespoons avocado oil

Salt and pepper (to taste)

1 cup baby spinach

Directions

In a medium saucepan bring 2 cups water to a boil. Add the potatoes and carrots and cook them for about 15 minutes or until soft.

Meanwhile, in a separate saucepan, boil 2 cups water and add in the eggs. Boil the eggs for about 10 minutes. Remove the eggs and immediately place in an ice bath for at least 3 minutes.

Once the potatoes and carrots are soft, drain the water and add in the avocado oil to the pot. Mash the carrots and potatoes together using a potato masher. Add the salt and pepper and set aside.

Divide the spinach between bowls and top with potato-carrot mash. Just before serving, peel a hard-boiled egg, slice, and top.

Notes

- *Storage (for leftovers or meal prep):* Refrigerate in an airtight container for up to 3 days.
- *Suggested additional toppings:* Add nuts and seeds or your favorite hot sauce.

○ ○ ◉ ○ ○

Scrambled Eggs with Peppers and Kale

1 serving • 15 minutes

Ingredients

¾ teaspoon extra virgin olive oil
½ red bell pepper, sliced
1 cup kale leaves, chopped

3 eggs
Sea salt and black pepper (to taste)

Directions

Heat the olive oil in a skillet over medium heat. Add the red bell pepper and kale leaves and sauté until softened, about 5 to 7 minutes.

While the veggies are cooking, crack the eggs into a bowl and season them with salt and pepper. Beat the eggs gently with a fork until well combined.

Push the veggies to one side of the pan, and pour the beaten eggs into the empty side. Use a spatula to scramble the eggs, slowly incorporating the veggies once the eggs are no longer very wet.

Divide between plates and enjoy.

Notes

- *Increase carbs:* Serve with toast, roasted potatoes, or sweet potatoes.
- *Make it vegan:* Use mashed tofu instead of eggs.

○ ○ ◉ ○ ○

Kale and Eggs

1 serving • 10 minutes

Ingredients

½ teaspoon ghee
3 cups kale leaves, roughly chopped
2 eggs
2 tablespoons pitted Kalamata olives
1 tablespoon nutritional yeast
⅛ teaspoon sea salt

Directions

Heat a skillet over medium heat and add the ghee. Add the kale and cook it for 2 to 3 minutes, until it's just wilted, stirring as needed.

Make two spaces in the kale and crack an egg into each space. Add the olives, and season everything with nutritional yeast and sea salt. Cover the skillet with a lid and cook the mixture for 3 to 4 minutes or until the eggs are cooked to your preference. Remove to a plate and enjoy!

Notes

- *Substitute ingredients:* Instead of kale, use another leafy green, such as collards, swiss chard, beet greens, or rapini. Instead of ghee, use organic butter, avocado oil, or olive oil.
- *Add flavor:* Add extra seasonings as desired to the kale, such as garlic.

○ ○ ◉ ○ ○

Soups and Salads

Cleaned-Up Chicken Salad

2 servings • 30 minutes

Ingredients

4 ounces cooked chicken breast (page 202), shredded
1 stalk celery, diced
¼ cup grapes, halved
2 cups kale leaves, finely sliced into ribbons
½ cup hemp hearts
2⅔ tablespoons slivered almonds
1 tablespoon Dijon mustard
1 tablespoon extra virgin olive oil
¼ lemon, juiced
Sea salt and black pepper (to taste)

Directions

Combine shredded chicken, celery, grapes, kale, hemp hearts, and slivered almonds to a bowl.

In a separate small bowl, whisk the mustard, olive oil, and lemon juice.

Add the dressing to the chicken mixture, and toss well to coat. Season with salt and pepper.

o o ◎ o o

Chicken, Kale, and Pepper Salad

1 serving • 15 minutes

Ingredients

1 red bell pepper, chopped
1 radish, sliced
1 avocado, sliced or cubed
½ cup kale leaves, thinly sliced
1 cup cooked quinoa (page 201)

4 ounces cooked chicken breast (page 202), chopped
2 tablespoons olive oil
2 tablespoons vinegar
Sea salt and black pepper (to taste)

Directions

Combine vegetables, quinoa, and chicken in a bowl. Toss with oil, vinegar, salt, and pepper.

o o ⊙ o o

Waldorf Salad with Chicken

2 servings • 15 minutes

Ingredients

3 stalks celery, chopped
4 ounces cooked chicken breast (page 202), chopped
1 apple, cored and chopped
5 leaves romaine, chopped

¼ cup toasted and chopped walnuts
3 tablespoons paleo mayonnaise
Salt and pepper (to taste)

Directions

In a bowl, toss together all ingredients.

o o ⊙ o o

Chicken, Pea, and Strawberry Salad

1 serving • 15 minutes

Ingredients

4 ounces cooked chicken breast (page 202), chopped

¼ cup fresh peas

¼ cup sliced strawberries

1 stalk green onion, chopped

1 cup mixed greens

2 tablespoons extra virgin olive oil

1 tablespoon balsamic vinegar

Directions

In a bowl, toss together all ingredients.

o o ◉ o o

Tofu Salad with Snow Peas

1 serving • 15 minutes

Ingredients

4 ounces firm tofu, cubed

½ cup snow peas, sliced

½ cup halved cherry tomatoes

1 cup mixed greens

½ avocado, diced

1 cup cooked quinoa (page 201)

2 tablespoons extra virgin olive oil

2 tablespoons soy sauce

Directions

In a bowl, toss together all ingredients.

o o ◉ o o

Salmon Salad with Avocado and Hearts of Palm

1 serving • 15 minutes

Ingredients

4 ounces cooked salmon fillet
(page 203), diced
1 avocado, diced
1 cup cooked quinoa (page 201)
1 can hearts of palm, sliced
½ cup cherry tomatoes, halved

½ cup kale leaves, sliced
2 tablespoons extra
virgin olive oil
1 tablespoon balsamic vinegar
Salt and pepper (to taste)

Directions

In a bowl, toss together all ingredients.

○ ○ ◉ ○ ○

Salmon and "Three Sisters" Salad

1 serving • 15 minutes

Ingredients

4 ounces cooked salmon fillet
(page 203)
¼ cup corn
¼ tomato, chopped
½ cup black beans
1 stalk green onion, chopped
2 tablespoons cilantro, chopped

½ avocado, chopped
1 cup mixed greens
2 tablespoons extra
virgin olive oil
1 tablespoon balsamic vinegar
Salt and pepper (to taste)

Directions

In a bowl, toss together all ingredients.

Notes

- *Substitute ingredient:* Instead of cilantro, use parsley.

○ ○ ◉ ○ ○

Herbed Chicken Salad with Grapes

1 serving • 15 minutes

Ingredients

4 ounces cooked chicken breast (page 202)

3 tablespoons paleo mayonnaise

2 stalks celery, chopped

½ cup grapes, halved

2 tablespoons fresh, chopped dill

Salt and pepper (to taste)

4 leaves romaine

Directions

In a bowl, toss together all ingredients except romaine. Divide mixture evenly atop romaine leaves.

Notes

- *Substitute ingredient:* Instead of dill, use tarragon.

○ ○ ◉ ○ ○

Italian-Style Lentil Soup

4 servings • 45 minutes

Ingredients

1 large red onion, diced

1 tablespoon chopped garlic

1 tablespoon extra virgin olive oil

1 cup dry red lentils

2 tablespoons tomato paste

1 quart organic chicken stock

1 tablespoon balsamic vinegar

1 teaspoon dried oregano

1 teaspoon sea salt

Directions

In a medium saucepan over medium-high heat, sauté the red onion and garlic in the olive oil until they have softened.

Add the red lentils and tomato paste to the pan and sauté for 1 minute.

Add the chicken stock, balsamic vinegar, oregano, and salt. Bring to a boil over high heat. Cover, reduce the heat to low, and simmer the soup for 30 minutes.

Use an immersion blender or carefully pour the soup into a standard blender and puree it until it's smooth. (If using a standard blender, remove the center cap from the lid and cover with a clean napkin to allow steam to vent. Blend carefully on low.)

○ ○ ◉ ○ ○

Chicken and Brown Rice Soup

4 servings • 30 minutes

Ingredients

1 quart organic chicken broth or stock

2 carrots, sliced

5 ounces cooked chicken breast (page 202), shredded

1 cup cooked brown rice (page 201)

¼ lemon

1 teaspoon fresh parsley, chopped, or to taste

Directions

Bring the chicken broth or stock to a boil, add the sliced carrots and simmer until the carrots have softened, about 8 minutes.

Add the chicken, rice, and a squeeze of lemon juice and stir lightly to combine.

Stir in fresh parsley before serving.

Notes

• *Substitute ingredient:* Instead of parsley, use dill.

○ ○ ◉ ○ ○

White Bean and Lemon Kale Soup

2 servings • 30 minutes

Ingredients

1½ cups organic vegetable broth, divided

1 carrot, chopped

1 leek (white parts only), finely chopped

1 clove garlic, minced

¼ teaspoon dried oregano

¾ teaspoon dried thyme

1 cup cooked cannellini beans, drained and rinsed

1½ cups water

2 cups kale leaves, stems removed, chopped

1½ tablespoons lemon juice

Sea salt and pepper (to taste)

2 tablespoons fresh chopped parsley

Directions

In a large pot over medium heat, add 2 tablespoons vegetable broth, carrots, and leeks. Cook the vegetables for 6 to 8 minutes, or until they are soft. Add the garlic, oregano, and thyme and cook for 1 to 2 minutes more.

Add the beans, 1½ cups water, and the remaining vegetable broth and bring the soup to a simmer over medium heat. Reduce the heat to medium-low and add the kale and lemon juice. Stir and continue cooking for 3 to 4 minutes, until the kale is wilted.

Season with salt and pepper. Ladle into bowls and top with parsley.

Notes

- *Storage (for leftovers or meal prep):* Refrigerate in an airtight container for up to 4 days.
- *Serving size:* One serving size is equal to about 1½ cups.
- *Suggested additional toppings:* Top with chili flakes and/or shredded parmesan.

○ ○ ◉ ○ ○

Recipe Staples

Quinoa

2 servings • 25 minutes

Ingredients

½ cup quinoa, uncooked

¾ cup water (plus water for rinsing)

Directions

Rinse uncooked quinoa thoroughly to clean, then drain. Combine the quinoa and ¾ cup water in a saucepan. Bring to a boil over high heat.

Reduce the heat to a simmer and cover the pan with a lid. Let it simmer for 13 to 15 minutes or until the water is absorbed. Remove the lid and fluff with a fork.

Notes

- *Storage (for leftovers or meal prep):* Refrigerate in an airtight container for up to 7 days.
- *Serving size:* ½ cup uncooked quinoa makes 1½ cups cooked quinoa.

○ ○ ◉ ○ ○

Brown Rice

2 servings • 15 minutes

Ingredients

½ cup brown rice, uncooked

1 cup water (plus water for rinsing)

Directions

Rinse uncooked rice thoroughly to clean, then drain. Repeat until water runs clear, then drain thoroughly.

Combine the rice and 1 cup water in a small pot. Bring to a boil over high heat.

Reduce the heat to a simmer and cover the pan with a lid. Let it simmer for 30 minutes or until the water is absorbed. Remove from heat and let sit, covered, for 10 more minutes. Remove the lid and fluff with a fork.

Notes

- *Storage (for leftovers or meal prep):* Refrigerate in an airtight container for up to 4 days.
- *Serving size:* ½ cup uncooked rice makes 1 cup cooked rice.

○ ○ ◉ ○ ○

Baked Chicken Breast

2 servings • 40 minutes

Ingredients

10 ounces chicken breast
(boneless, skinless)

1 tablespoon extra virgin olive oil

¼ teaspoon salt

Directions

Preheat oven to 400°F (204°C). Line a baking dish with parchment paper.

Place chicken breasts in the prepared baking dish. Drizzle with oil and season with salt, rubbing evenly over both sides of the chicken. Bake for about 25 to 30 minutes, or until the chicken is cooked through. (The center must reach 160°F.)

Remove the chicken from the oven and let rest in the dish, covered with a piece of aluminum foil, for at least 10 minutes.

Carefully remove the foil and slice the chicken before serving. Enjoy!

Notes

- *Storage (for leftovers or meal prep):* Refrigerate in an airtight container for up to 4 days.
- *Add flavor:* If not making for another recipe, try adding seasonings such as chili powder, garlic powder, or other dried herbs.

○ ○ ◉ ○ ○

Baked Salmon

2 servings • 15 minutes

Ingredients

10-ounce salmon fillet

1 tablespoon extra virgin olive oil

¼ teaspoon salt

½ teaspoon ground black pepper

Directions

Preheat oven to 450°F (232°C). Line a baking dish with parchment paper.

Place the salmon fillets on the prepared baking sheet. Drizzle with oil and season with sea salt and black pepper, rubbing evenly over both sides of the fish.

Bake the salmon in the oven for 15 minutes, or until it is opaque and flakes easily with a fork.

Notes

- *Storage (for leftovers or meal prep):* Refrigerate in an airtight container for up to 4 days.
- *Add flavor:* If not making for another recipe, try adding seasonings such as dill and lemon, garlic powder, or other dried herbs

○ ○ ◉ ○ ○

Mains and Sides

Sweet Potato "Toasts" with Salmon, Avocado, and Salsa

1 serving • 15 minutes

Ingredients

1 sweet potato

1 avocado, mashed

4 ounces cooked salmon fillet (page 203), diced

¼ cup organic salsa

Directions

Peel sweet potato and slice lengthwise into ¼- or ⅓-inch slices. Place in toaster on high setting until desired doneness (may take two or three cycles, depending on your toaster).

Top the sweet potato "toasts" with the mashed avocado, diced salmon, and salsa.

Notes

- *Tip:* Instead of using a toaster, bake the sweet potato slices on a parchment-lined baking sheet in your oven at 350°F (175°C) for 15 minutes or until desired doneness.

o o ◉ o o

Chicken Lettuce Tacos

1 serving • 15 minutes

Ingredients

4 ounces cooked chicken breast
(page 202), diced

1 avocado, diced

1 red bell pepper, diced

4 romaine lettuce leaves

¼ cup organic salsa

½ cup cooked quinoa (page 201)

Directions

Evenly divide the chicken, avocado, and bell pepper onto the romaine leaves. Roll each tightly into a "taco."

Top each taco with salsa, and serve with a side of quinoa.

Notes

- *Substitute ingredient:* Instead of quinoa, serve with brown rice (see page 201).

○ ○ ◉ ○ ○

Salmon-Stuffed Avocados

2 servings • 15 minutes

Ingredients

1 avocado, halved

4 ounces cooked salmon fillet (page 203), chopped

¼ cup organic salsa

1 cup mixed greens, roughly chopped

2 tablespoons extra virgin olive oil

1 tablespoon balsamic vinegar

Salt and pepper, to taste

½ cup cooked brown rice (page 201)

Directions

Top each avocado half with chopped salmon and salsa.

Toss the mixed greens with the olive oil, balsamic vinegar, and salt and pepper. Divide onto two plates.

Serve one salmon-stuffed avocado atop each plate of mixed greens with a side of brown rice.

○ ○ ◉ ○ ○

Tofu with Veggies and Brown Rice

1 serving • 15 minutes

Ingredients

4 ounces extra-firm tofu, sliced

Salt and pepper, to taste

1 cup cooked brown rice (page 201)

½ cup steamed broccoli

1 red bell pepper, sliced

2 teaspoons soy sauce

Juice of ½ lime

Directions

Sprinkle the tofu slices with salt and pepper and place on a microwave-safe plate, alongside the brown rice; microwave on high until warm. Serve with steamed broccoli and sliced fresh bell peppers. Drizzle with soy sauce and a squeeze of lime.

○ ○ ◉ ○ ○

Japanese Tofu Bowls

1 serving • 15 minutes

Ingredients

½ sweet potato

1 cup cooked brown rice (page 201), served cold

4 ounces extra-firm tofu, chopped

½ avocado, diced

½ cucumber, sliced

1 cup steamed mixed greens

1 tablespoon soy sauce

Directions

Peel sweet potato and slice lengthwise into ¼- or ⅓-inch slices. Place in toaster on high setting until desired doneness (may take two or three cycles, depending on your toaster).

Spoon the brown rice into a serving bowl. Top the rice with the tofu, avocado, cucumber, sweet potato "toasts," and steamed greens. Drizzle with soy sauce.

Notes

- *Tip:* Instead of using a toaster, bake the sweet potato slices on a parchment-lined baking sheet in your oven at 350°F (175°C) for 15 minutes or until desired doneness.

o o ◉ o o

One-Pan Salmon with Green Beans and Roasted Tomato

2 servings • 25 minutes

Ingredients

2 cups green beans, washed and trimmed

1 cup cherry tomatoes, whole

1½ teaspoon extra virgin olive oil

Sea salt and black pepper, to taste

10-ounce salmon fillet

Directions

Preheat the oven to 510°F (266°C).

Place the green beans and cherry tomatoes in a mixing bowl and toss them with the olive oil until they are evenly coated. Season with sea salt and black pepper to taste and toss again. Transfer them to a baking sheet and bake them for 10 minutes.

Season the salmon fillets with sea salt and black pepper, to taste.

Remove the baking sheet from the oven and place the salmon fillets on top of the veggies. Place the sheet back in the oven and bake for 7 to 10 minutes or until salmon is opaque and flakes easily with a fork.

Divide the veggies between two plates and top with salmon.

Notes

- *Substitute ingredients:* Instead of salmon, use any type of fish fillet. Baking times will vary depending on thickness. Instead of olive oil, use coconut oil.
- *Make it vegan:* Use roasted chickpeas instead of salmon. Drain and rinse 1 can of chickpeas. Add them in with the green beans and tomatoes, and bake as instructed.
- *Increase carbs:* Serve with quinoa or rice (see page 201).
- *Serving suggestion:* Drizzle balsamic vinegar over the veggies before serving.

○ ○ ◉ ○ ○

Salsa Verde Salmon with Tomatoes and Brown Rice

2 servings • 45 minutes

Ingredients

½ cup uncooked brown rice

2 tablespoons extra virgin olive oil, divided

10-ounce salmon fillet

2 cups cherry tomatoes, halved

½ teaspoon sea salt

1 tablespoon capers

¼ cup fresh parsley, finely chopped

1 tablespoon apple cider vinegar

Directions

Cook the brown rice according to the directions on the package, or follow recipe on page 201.

About 15 minutes before the rice is done cooking, heat half the olive oil in a large pan over medium-high heat. Add the salmon and tomatoes, season with salt. Cook the salmon for 3 to 5 minutes each side, or until it is opaque and flakes easily with a fork.

Meanwhile, in a small bowl, combine the capers, parsley, vinegar, and remaining olive oil. Mix well.

Divide the brown rice onto plates and top it with the salmon, tomatoes, and the caper-parsley salsa verde.

Notes

- *Storage (for leftovers or meal prep):* Keeps well in the fridge for 2 to 3 days.
- *Substitute ingredients:* Instead of brown rice, use basmati rice, jasmine rice, quinoa, couscous, or cauliflower rice. Instead of capers, use olives.
- *Tip:* Cook the rice beforehand to save time. You will need 1 cup of cooked brown rice for this recipe (see page 201).

○ ○ ◉ ○ ○

Turkey and Carrots with Spinach

4 servings • 25 minutes

Ingredients

2 cups water

4 carrots, peeled and chopped

2 tablespoons avocado oil, divided

1 pound extra-lean ground turkey

8 cups baby spinach

1 tablespoon nutritional yeast

Directions

Bring 2 cups water to a boil in a medium saucepan. Add the carrots and cook them for 10 minutes or until they are soft. Drain the carrots and set them aside.

While the carrots cook, heat half the avocado oil in a separate pan over medium heat, then add the ground turkey. Use a spatula to break up the meat as it browns. Cook the turkey for 8 to 10 minutes, until no pink remains. Once it's cooked, drain the fat and set the meat aside.

In the same pan, add in the other half of the avocado oil and the spinach. Sauté the spinach over medium heat until wilted, about 2 to 3 minutes. Season with the nutritional yeast.

Divide the turkey, carrots, and spinach evenly.

Notes

- *Storage (for leftovers or meal prep):* Refrigerate in an airtight container for up to 3 days.
- *Substitute ingredient:* Instead of spinach, use another leafy green like Swiss chard or kale.
- *Make it vegan:* Use cooked black beans or lentils instead of ground turkey.

○ ○ ◉ ○ ○

Cold Salmon Bowls with Sweet Potato "Toasts"

1 serving • 20 minutes

Ingredients

1 sweet potato

½ cup cooked brown rice, served cold (page 201)

4 ounces cooked salmon fillet (page 203), chopped and served cold

1 avocado, chopped

¼ cucumber, chopped

1 teaspoon soy sauce

Directions

Peel sweet potato and slice lengthwise into ¼- or ⅓-inch slices. Place in toaster on high setting until desired doneness (may take two or three cycles, depending on your toaster).

Spoon the brown rice into a serving bowl.

Top the rice with chopped salmon, avocado, cucumber, and some sweet potato. Drizzle with soy sauce.

Notes

- *Make it vegan:* Substitute the salmon with 4 ounces extra-firm tofu, chopped.
- *Tip:* Instead of using a toaster, bake the sweet potato slices on a parchment-lined baking sheet in your oven at 350°F (175°C) for 15 minutes or until desired doneness.

○ ○ ◉ ○ ○

Mediterranean-Style Crispy Tofu

2 servings • 25 minutes (plus optional 24-hour marinade)

Ingredients

2 tablespoons extra virgin olive oil, divided

1½ teaspoon fresh crushed garlic

1 teaspoon dried oregano

½ teaspoon dried thyme

½ teaspoon sea salt

½ teaspoon black pepper

1 lemon, halved, divided

½ block (8 ounces) firm tofu, cubed

2 cups baby kale leaves

½ cup cooked brown rice (page 201)

½ orange bell pepper, chopped

½ small head broccoli, steamed

½ avocado, cubed

2 tablespoons hummus

Directions

In a medium-sized airtight container, add 1 tablespoon olive oil, garlic, herbs, salt, pepper, and juice from half the lemon. Whisk until well combined.

Add in the tofu cubes, put the lid on the container, and shake it gently until the cubes are nicely coated with your marinade. Marinate the tofu for at least 15 minutes. (See tip.)

Remove tofu from marinade and gently pat with paper towels to remove excess marinade. In a large nonstick pan, heat 1 tablespoon of olive oil on medium-high heat. Fry the tofu, rotating them gently to ensure all the sides have a crispy coating.

Place the tofu cubes on a plate lined with paper towels to soak up any excess oil. Set aside.

Fill the base of two bowls with baby kale, followed by ¼ cup of brown rice each. Divide the peppers, broccoli, and avocado between the bowls. Top each bowl with 1 tablespoon of hummus and the crispy tofu cubes. Finish with the juice of the rest of the lemon. Serve immediately.

Notes

- *Tip:* For the best flavor, allow the tofu to marinate for 24 hours.

○ ○ ◎ ○ ○

Sweet Potato "Toasts" with Chicken and Hummus

1 serving • 15 minutes

Ingredients

1 sweet potato

¼ cup plain hummus

4 ounces cooked chicken breast (page 202), shredded

¼ cup organic salsa

½ cup cooked brown rice (page 201)

Directions

Peel sweet potato and slice lengthwise into ¼- or ⅓-inch slices. Place in toaster on high setting until desired doneness (may take two or three cycles, depending on your toaster).

Let the sweet potato "toasts" cool a bit and then top with the hummus, chicken, and salsa. Serve with brown rice on the side.

Notes

- *Substitute ingredient:* Use quinoa instead of brown rice.
- *Tip:* Instead of using a toaster, bake the sweet potato slices on a parchment-lined baking sheet in your oven at 350°F (175°C) for 15 minutes or until desired doneness.

○ ○ ◉ ○ ○

PREBIOTIC RECIPES

Banana and Blueberry Quinoa Porridge

3 servings • 25 minutes

Ingredients

½ cup dry tricolor quinoa, rinsed and drained

1½ cups nondairy milk, divided

½ cup water

¼ teaspoon cinnamon

⅛ teaspoon sea salt

1 small banana, mashed

1½ cups blueberries

¼ cup hemp seeds

Directions

Add the quinoa, 1¼ cups of the nondairy milk, ½ cup water, the cinnamon, and the salt to a pot. Bring to a boil.

Reduce heat to low, cover the pot, and simmer until the liquid has been absorbed and the quinoa is tender but still chewy, about 15 minutes.

Remove the pot from the heat and let stand for 5 minutes. Fluff the quinoa with a fork and fold in the mashed banana.

Divide the porridge evenly between bowls and serve it topped with the blueberries, hemp seeds, and the remaining milk.

Notes

- *Storage (for leftovers or meal prep):* Refrigerate in an airtight container for up to 3 days.
- *Serving size:* One serving size is equal to approximately ½ cup quinoa.
- *Suggested additional toppings:* Use strawberries, raspberries, and/or blackberries.
- *Substitute ingredient:* Use pumpkin seeds, sunflower seeds, and/or chia seeds instead of hemp seeds.
- *Tip:* The quinoa can be prepared ahead of time and stored in the refrigerator. Reheat it on the stove or in the microwave when ready to serve.

○ ○ ◉ ○ ○

Almond and Oat Breakfast Cookies

12 servings • 20 minutes

Ingredients

1 medium banana, mashed

1 egg

½ cup almond butter (runny)

⅓ cup maple syrup

1 teaspoon vanilla extract

1½ cups rolled oats

1 teaspoon baking powder

¼ cup hemp seeds

2 tablespoons chia seeds

¼ teaspoon sea salt

Directions

Preheat the oven to 350°F (175°C). Line a baking sheet with parchment paper.

In a large bowl, add the banana, egg, almond butter, maple syrup, and vanilla. Stir until well combined.

Add the oats, baking powder, hemp seeds, chia seeds, and salt. Mix with a spatula until combined.

Using clean and slightly damp hands, or a cookie scoop, form the dough into 12 large cookies, about 2 tablespoons per cookie, and place them on the baking sheet.

Bake the cookies for 14 minutes, or until they are golden brown.

Allow them to cool on the baking sheet for 5 minutes before moving them to a cooling rack.

Notes

- *Storage (for leftovers or meal prep):* Store in an airtight container at room temperature for up to 2 days. Refrigerate or freeze if storing longer.
- *Make it vegan:* Replace the egg with a flax egg.
- *Add flavor:* Add cinnamon with the dry ingredients, to taste.
- *Tip:* The dough is sticky, so using a medium cookie scoop or a small ice cream scoop is easier than using your hands.

○ ○ ◉ ○ ○

Salmon, Veggie, and Egg Bowl

2 servings • 30 minutes

Ingredients

1 cup mini potatoes (halved)

1 tablespoon avocado
oil, divided

Sea salt and black
pepper, to taste

8-ounce salmon fillet

2 cups bok choy, finely chopped

2 tablespoons water

4 eggs

2 tablespoons sauerkraut

Directions

Preheat the oven to 400°F (205°C). Add the potatoes to a baking sheet. Toss them with ⅓ of the oil, and salt and pepper to taste.

Bake the potatoes for 15 minutes. Remove the sheet from the oven, toss the potatoes, and add the salmon fillet to the same baking sheet. Bake for 15 minutes or until the potatoes are tender and the salmon is cooked through.

While the potatoes and salmon are baking, heat the remaining oil in a pan over medium heat. Add the bok choy, cook it for 1 minute while stirring. Add 2 tablespoons water, and cook the bok choy for 5 more minutes, stirring occasionally. Remove bok choy from pan.

Crack the eggs into a bowl and beat gently with a fork until well combined. Add the eggs to the pan and scramble them until they reach desired doneness.

Evenly divide the potatoes, salmon, eggs, and bok choy between two bowls. Top with 1 tablespoon sauerkraut each.

Notes

- *Storage (for leftovers or meal prep):* Refrigerate in an airtight container for up to 3 days.
- *Add flavor:* Add 1 teaspoon garlic powder and ¼ cup onions to potatoes.
- *Suggested additional toppings:* Add microgreens.

○ ○ ◎ ○ ○

Soups and Salads

Farro and Beet Salad

2 servings • 30 minutes

Ingredients

½ cup uncooked farro, rinsed

4 medium beets, cubed in small pieces

2 cloves garlic

1 cup vegetable broth, divided

Sea salt and black pepper, to taste

½ small lemon, juiced and zested

¼ cup fresh chopped dill

1 cup microgreens

Directions

Cook the farro according to the package directions. Set aside to cool.

Meanwhile, preheat the oven to 425°F (220°C) and line a rimmed baking sheet with parchment paper.

Place the beets and unpeeled garlic on the baking sheet. Drizzle with ¾ cup of the broth and season with salt and pepper to taste. Toss to coat the beets and garlic and spread the veggies in a single layer. Bake them, flipping them once halfway through cooking, until the beets are tender, about 15 to 18 minutes. Set aside to cool.

Peel the cooked garlic cloves and mash them in a small bowl with the remaining broth, lemon zest, and lemon juice.

Add the garlic mixture, beets, dill, and microgreens to the farro. Stir until combined and serve.

Notes

- *Storage (for leftovers or meal prep):* Refrigerate in an airtight container for up to 3 days.
- *Add flavor:* Use extra virgin olive oil instead of broth.
- *Suggested additional toppings:* Add chives, parsley, and/or basil leaves before mixing the salad. Top it with goat or feta cheese and/or pumpkin or sunflower seeds.

○ ○ ◉ ○ ○

Celery Root and Carrot Chicken Salad

4 servings • 40 minutes

Ingredients

10-ounce chicken breast (boneless, skinless)
2 cups celery root, shredded
2 medium carrots, shredded
1 tablespoon sesame oil
1 tablespoon rice vinegar
½ teaspoon garlic powder
1 tablespoon fresh grated ginger
1 teaspoon sea salt

Directions

Preheat the oven to 375°F (190°C). Line a baking sheet with parchment paper.

Place the chicken breast(s) on a baking sheet and bake them for 30 minutes.

Meanwhile, combine the celery root and carrots to a large mixing bowl. Once the chicken is done, shred it with two forks and add it to the celery root and carrot mixture.

Add the sesame oil, rice vinegar, garlic powder, grated ginger, and salt to the bowl. Toss to coat the salad and transfer it to serving bowls.

Notes

- *Storage (for leftovers or meal prep):* Refrigerate in an airtight container for up to 3 days.
- *Serving size:* One serving is equal to approximately 1½ cups.
- *Suggested additional toppings:* Add shredded purple cabbage, green or red onions, raisins, honey, or maple syrup.
- *Serving suggestion:* Enjoy as is, over a bed of lettuce, in a sandwich, or in a tortilla as a wrap.

○ ○ ◉ ○ ○

Curried Potato and Pea Stew

2 servings • 1 hour

Ingredients

6 cups vegetable broth, divided
1 small white onion, diced
3 cloves garlic, minced
1 cup dried green peas
2 cups chopped mini potatoes

1 teaspoon madras curry powder
Sea salt and black pepper, to taste
2 tablespoons fresh, chopped cilantro (optional)

Directions

Add a splash of the vegetable broth to a large pot over medium heat. Add the onion, stir, and cook for 2 to 3 minutes or until softened. Add the garlic and cook for 2 to 3 minutes.

Add the dried green peas and the remaining broth. Bring it to a boil for 10 minutes, then reduce the heat to low, cover the pot with a lid, and simmer the stew for 15 minutes.

Add the potatoes, curry powder, salt, and pepper. Continue to simmer the stew for another 20 minutes, or until it has thickened and most of the liquid has reduced.

Divide evenly between bowls. Top with cilantro.

Notes

- *Storage (for leftovers or meal prep):* Refrigerate in an airtight container for up to 5 days. Freeze for up to 3 months.
- *Serving size:* One serving is equal to approximately 2 cups.
- *Suggested additional toppings:* Add microgreens and/or hemp seeds.
- *Substitute ingredient:* Instead of dried green peas, use split green or yellow peas instead and reduce the cooking time.

○ ○ ◉ ○ ○

Edamame Potato Soup

2 servings • 30 minutes

Ingredients

1½ cups vegetable broth
½ medium yellow
onion, chopped
2 yellow potatoes,
peeled and diced
¼ ounce thyme sprigs

1 cup frozen edamame (thawed,
plus extra for optional garnish)
Sea salt and black
pepper, to taste
½ lemon, juiced

Directions

Add the vegetable broth, onion, potatoes, and thyme sprigs to a pot. Bring the soup to a boil, then reduce the heat to simmer. Cover the pot with a lid and let the soup simmer for 15 to 20 minutes or until the potatoes are soft.

Add the edamame to the pot and let the soup simmer covered for another 5 minutes. Season with salt and pepper, to taste.

Remove the thyme sprigs from the pot. Use an immersion blender or carefully pour the soup into a standard blender. Puree the soup until it is smooth.

Stir in the lemon juice. Divide the soup evenly between bowls. If desired, top with more edamame before enjoying.

Notes

- *Storage (for leftovers or meal prep):* Refrigerate in an airtight container for up to 3 days.
- *Serving size:* One serving is equal to approximately 2 cups.
- *Add flavor:* Add cumin, chili flakes, and garlic powder, to taste.

○ ○ ◉ ○ ○

Mains and Sides

Roasted Jerusalem Artichokes with Pomegranate and Sage

2 servings • 30 minutes

Ingredients

1½ cups Jerusalem artichokes, trimmed and halved

1 tablespoon extra virgin olive oil

1 teaspoon dried rosemary

Sea salt and black pepper, to taste)

2 tablespoons pomegranate seeds

1 tablespoon fresh sage

Directions

Preheat the oven to 400°F (205°C).

Toss the Jerusalem artichokes with the oil, rosemary, salt, and pepper. Add them to a cast-iron pan or oven-safe dish.

Roast the artichokes for 20 minutes, tossing them halfway through. They should be tender and slightly browned.

Top with pomegranate seeds and fresh sage.

Notes

- *Storage (for leftovers or meal prep):* Refrigerate in an airtight container and consume within 3 days. The Jerusalem artichokes will start to brown within 1 day, but they are still edible.
- *Serving size:* One serving size is about ¾ cup.
- *Add flavor:* Add minced garlic and/or shallot before roasting.

○ ○ ◎ ○ ○

One Pan Salmon, Beans, and Potatoes

4 servings • 35 minutes

Ingredients

2½ cups chopped mini potatoes

1½ cups frozen corn

1½ cups frozen green beans

2 tablespoons coconut aminos, divided

⅛ ounce avocado oil spray

½ teaspoon black pepper

1 pound salmon fillets

Directions

Preheat the oven to 400°F (205°C). Spread the potatoes, corn, and green beans evenly on a baking sheet. Toss with 1 tablespoon of coconut aminos. Spray with the avocado oil and season with black pepper. Bake the veggies for 15 minutes.

Remove the baking sheet and add the salmon fillets. Top with the remaining coconut aminos and bake for another 15 minutes or until cooked through. Divide evenly between plates.

Notes

- *Storage (for leftovers or meal prep):* Refrigerate in an airtight container for up to 3 days.
- *Add flavor:* Add garlic powder and onion powder to taste.
- *Substitute ingredient:* Insetad of coconut aminos, use tamari or soy sauce.
- *Tip:* One-eighth ounce of avocado oil spray is equal to a one-second spray.

○ ○ ◉ ○ ○

Za'atar Roasted Beets and Eggplant

3 servings • 35 minutes

Ingredients

½ medium eggplant, chopped

2 medium beets,
peeled and cubed

2 teaspoons extra virgin olive oil

2 tablespoons za'atar spice

1 tablespoon fresh,
chopped parsley

1 tablespoon hemp seeds

Directions

Preheat the oven to 375°F (190°C). Line a baking sheet with parchment paper.

Toss the eggplant, beets, olive oil, and za'atar spice together in a bowl. Spread the vegetables out on the baking sheet and roast them for 25 to 30 minutes or until the edges are brown and starting to get crispy.

Add the vegetables to serving bowls and garnish with parsley and hemp seeds.

Notes

- *Storage (for leftovers or meal prep):* Refrigerate in an airtight container for up to 3 days.
- *Serving size:* One serving is ¾ cup.
- *Add flavor:* Add garlic and/or shallots to the vegetables before roasting them. Plate the vegetables on top of hummus for added creaminess.
- *Suggested additional toppings:* Add dried cranberries or chopped, pitted dates.

○ ○ ◉ ○ ○

One-Pan Sausage, Turnip, and Jerusalem Artichokes

4 servings • 30 minutes

Ingredients

2 tablespoons unsalted butter

2 cups Jerusalem artichokes, chopped

2 medium turnips, chopped

1 pound chicken sausage, chopped

Sea salt and black pepper, to taste

2 tablespoons fresh, chopped sage

Directions

Melt the butter in a large pan over medium heat. Add the Jerusalem artichokes and cook them for 10 minutes, stirring frequently.

Add the turnips and cook for another 5 minutes.

Add the chicken sausage and continue to cook for 7 to 10 minutes, until the Jerusalem artichokes and turnip are fork tender and the sausage is cooked through. Season with salt, pepper, and sage.

Notes

- *Storage (for leftovers or meal prep):* Refrigerate in an airtight container for up to 3 days.
- *Serving size:* One serving is equal to approximately 1¼ cups.
- *Add flavor:* Add garlic and onions.
- *Suggested additional toppings:* Add fried eggs.
- *Make it vegan:* Use tempeh or plant-based sausage instead of chicken sausage. Use coconut, olive, or avocado oil in place of the butter.

o o ◉ o o

PROBIOTIC RECIPES

Blueberry Coconut Kefir Oatmeal

2 servings • 5 minutes

Ingredients

⅔ cup quick oats

1 tablespoon chia seeds

1 teaspoon cinnamon

1⅓ cup plain kefir

¾ cup blueberries (fresh or frozen)

1 tablespoon unsweetened shredded coconut

Directions

In a jar or mixing bowl, combine the oats, chia seeds, cinnamon, and kefir. Divide into bowls and top with blueberries and shredded coconut.

Notes

- *Storage (for leftovers or meal prep):* Refrigerate in an airtight container for up to 5 days.
- *Serving size:* One serving is equal to approximately 1½ cups.
- *Make it gluten-free:* Use gluten-free oats. (While oats are naturally gluten-free, you must buy a product with a "gluten-free" label to ensure that they're processed and packaged in a gluten-free facility and tested to meet FDA standards for gluten-free designation.)
- *Make it vegan or dairy-free:* Use coconut yogurt instead of kefir.
- *Suggested additional toppings:* Add maple syrup, honey, nutmeg, nuts, nut butter, hemp seeds, dark chocolate chips, raisins, or fruit.

o o ⊙ o o

Kefir Berry Smoothie

1 serving • 5 minutes

Ingredients

1½ cup frozen berries
1 cup plain kefir
½ medium banana

1 tablespoon sunflower seed butter

Directions

Place all ingredients in a blender and blend until smooth. Pour into a glass.

Notes

- *Make it vegan and dairy-free:* Use coconut yogurt instead of kefir.
- *Substitute ingredient:* Instead of sunflower seed butter, use almond or peanut butter.
- *Increase the sweetness:* Add maple syrup, honey, or dates, to taste.

○ ○ ◉ ○ ○

Tempeh and Arugula Benedict

2 servings • 35 minutes

Ingredients

8 ounces tempeh (cut into 2 x 2-inch squares)
1 large sweet potato, cut into rounds
2 tablespoons extra virgin olive oil, divided
¼ cup cashews (raw, soaked for at least 6 hours, drained and rinsed)
1 tablespoon lemon juice
¼ teaspoon turmeric

½ teaspoon sea salt
¼ cup water
1 cup arugula

Directions

Preheat the oven to 375°F (190°C). Brush both sides of the tempeh squares and sweet potato rounds with half the olive oil. Place them on a baking sheet and bake them for 30 minutes, or until the sweet potatoes are fork-tender.

Add the remaining olive oil, cashews, lemon juice, turmeric, salt, and ¼ cup water to a blender. Blend for approximately 1 minute, or until smooth and creamy. Add a little more water if necessary to achieve your desired consistency.

Stack the sweet potato rounds, arugula, and tempeh, then drizzle on the cashew hollandaise!

Notes

- *Storage (for leftovers or meal prep):* Refrigerate in an airtight container for up to 5 days. Ingredients are best kept separately before serving.
- *Serving size:* One serving is equal to 2 sweet potato rounds, 2 pieces of tempeh, ½ cup arugula, and approximately ¼ cup of cashew hollandaise.
- *Add flavor:* Add garlic powder or smoked paprika to the hollandaise. Use smoked tempeh.
- *Suggested additional toppings:* Add microgreens or tomato slices.
- *Tip:* Soak the cashews in boiling water for 10 minutes to reduce soaking time.

○ ○ ◉ ○ ○

Mains and Sides

Kimchi

8 servings • 30 minutes

Ingredients

4 cups green cabbage (tightly packed)

6 stalks green onion, diced

1 large carrot, grated

1 cup grated radishes (about 1 small bunch)

4 cloves garlic, minced

3 tablespoons fresh grated ginger (peeled)

1 tablespoon sea salt

1 tablespoon red pepper flakes

Directions

Core and finely slice your cabbage. Place the cabbage in a mixing bowl with all other ingredients. Using clean hands, massage the salt into the cabbage and vegetables until it starts to soften (5 to 10 minutes). Set the bowl aside and let the mixture rest for 10 minutes, then massage it again for another 5 minutes.

Transfer the kimchi into sterilized jars, leaving an inch of space at the top. Pack it down into the jar until the brine rises to cover the vegetables. Seal the jars with sterilized lids.

Let the kimchi ferment at room temperature for 3 to 5 days. It may bubble, and that is normal. Check on your kimchi every day and resubmerge the vegetables under the brine if they rise.

Taste your kimchi on day 3. If it tastes ripe, transfer it to the fridge. If not, let it ferment another day or two.

Enjoy your kimchi right away or let it sit for another week or two for extra flavor.

Notes

- *Serving suggestion:* Serve it with burgers, salads, or in our Kimchi Jackfruit Bowls (see page 229).

○ ○ ◉ ○ ○

Kimchi Jackfruit Bowls

3 servings • 40 minutes

Ingredients

½ cup brown rice, uncooked

1¾ cups canned young jackfruit, drained and rinsed

1 clove garlic, minced

1½ tablespoons tamari

1 teaspoon coconut sugar

¼ teaspoon red pepper flakes

¼ lime, juiced

1 teaspoon sesame oil

1 cucumber, diced

2 medium carrots, grated or diced

½ cup kimchi (from the recipe on page 228 or store-bought)

1 tablespoon sesame seeds

1 stalk green onion, diced

Directions

Cook brown rice according to package directions or recipe on page 201.

In a pan over medium heat, add the jackfruit, garlic, tamari, coconut sugar, red pepper flakes, and lime juice. Stir well until combined and use a spatula to break up and shred the jackfruit. Cook for 15 minutes, or until the jackfruit is soft. Once it is done, add the sesame oil and remove the pan from the heat.

Plate the rice, and add the cucumber, carrots, kimchi, and jackfruit. Top with sesame seeds and diced green onion.

Notes

- *Storage (for leftovers or meal prep):* Store ingredients separately in airtight containers in the fridge for 3 to 5 days. Reheat the jackfruit mix before serving.
- *Make it grain-free:* Serve over mixed greens or cauliflower rice instead of brown rice.
- *Substitute ingredient:* Instead of tamari, use soy sauce or coconut aminos.
- *Tip:* Cook the rice beforehand to save time. You will need 1½ cups cooked brown rice for this recipe.

○ ○ ◉ ○ ○

Goat Cheese Zucchini Rolls

1 serving • 10 minutes

Ingredients

¼ cup goat cheese, crumbled

1 zucchini, ends trimmed and thinly sliced length-wise

Directions

Slice the zucchini so that the pieces are flexible enough to roll without breaking.

Spread a thin layer of goat cheese on each slice of zucchini.

Gently roll them into small pinwheels.

Notes

- *Storage (for leftovers or meal prep):* Refrigerate in an airtight container for up to 3 days.
- *Serving size:* One zucchini makes approximately 12 rolls.
- *Make it vegan and dairy-free:* Use cashew cream cheese instead.
- *Add flavor:* Mix your choice of fresh herbs into the goat cheese. Drizzle the goat cheese with extra virgin olive oil before rolling the pinwheels.

○ ○ ◉ ○ ○

Fresh Figs and Goat Milk Yogurt

1 serving • 5 minutes

Ingredients

½ cup plain goat milk yogurt

1 fig, sliced

Directions

Add the yogurt to a bowl and top with the sliced fig.

Notes

- *Storage (for leftovers or meal prep):* Refrigerate in an airtight container and consume within 1 day.
- *Suggested additional toppings:* Drizzle with honey and/or top with chopped walnuts, pecans, sunflower seeds, hemp seeds, or cacao nibs.

o o ⊙ o o

Apple, Brie, and Sauerkraut Bites

2 servings • 10 minutes

Ingredients

1 apple

3 ounces Brie

¼ cup sauerkraut

Directions

Slice the apple horizontally into rounds. Slice the Brie into thin slices of about the same size as the apple rounds.

Stack the apple rounds with the Brie and sauerkraut.

Notes

- *Storage (for leftovers or meal prep):* Best enjoyed immediately but may be refrigerated in an airtight container for up to 2 days.
- *Make it vegan or dairy-free:* Use vegan cheese in place of the Brie.
- *Suggested additional toppings:* Drizzle each bite with a balsamic reduction or honey.

o o ⊙ o o

Tempeh Patties

4 servings • 20 minutes

Ingredients

8 ounces tempeh, cubed

1 small yellow onion, diced

2 garlic cloves, peeled

1 teaspoon chili powder

½ teaspoon dried parsley

½ teaspoon paprika

Sea salt and black pepper, to taste

1 tablespoon coconut aminos

2 tablespoons extra virgin olive oil, divided

Directions

Add the tempeh, onion, garlic, chili powder, parsley, paprika, salt, pepper, coconut aminos, and 1 tablespoon of olive oil into a food processor. Pulse until everything is combined and resembles a sausage-like texture.

Form the mixture into equal balls then flatten them to approximately 1-inch-thick patties.

Heat the remaining oil in a pan over medium heat. Add the patties and cook for 3 to 5 minutes per side or until they are golden brown.

Notes

- *Storage (for leftovers or meal prep):* Refrigerate in an airtight container for up to 3 days.
- *Serving size:* One serving is 1 patty.
- *Serving suggestion:* Enjoy as is or alongside potatoes, hash browns, or as part of a breakfast sandwich.

○ ○ ◎ ○ ○

Spicy Miso Steak

4 servings • 15 minutes

Ingredients

12-ounce New York strip steak

Sea salt and black pepper, to taste

2 tablespoons extra virgin olive oil, divided

2 tablespoons miso paste

¼ cup water

¼ cup sriracha

1 tablespoon honey

2 stalks green onion, thinly sliced

Directions

Season the steak with salt and pepper.

In a pan over medium-high heat, add 1 tablespoon olive oil. Cook the steak for 3 to 4 minutes per side, or until it reaches your desired doneness. Set steak aside, and let rest while preparing rest of meal.

Reduce the temperature to medium-low. In the same pan, whisk in the remaining oil, miso, ¼ cup water, sriracha, and honey. Once combined, remove sauce from heat.

Slice the steak, and divide evenly between 4 plates. Drizzle each with the spicy miso sauce, and garnish with green onions.

Notes

- *Storage (for leftovers or meal prep):* Refrigerate in an airtight container for up to 4 days.
- *Add flavor:* Add more honey for a sweeter sauce. For less spice, reduce the amount of sriracha sauce.
- *Substitute ingredient:* If spice is not tolerated, substitute tomato sauce for the sriracha.

o o ⊙ o o

Coconut Yogurt Tofu

4 servings • 20 minutes (plus optional overnight marinade)

Ingredients

1 cup unsweetened
coconut yogurt

1⅔ tablespoons taco seasoning

1 teaspoon sea salt, to taste

1 block (16 ounces) extra-firm
tofu, pressed and sliced

1 tablespoon extra virgin olive
oil, divided

8 cups baby spinach

Directions

In a bowl, combine the coconut yogurt, taco seasoning, and salt. Add the tofu slices and coat them well in the mixture.

Heat 1 teaspoon olive oil in a nonstick skillet over medium heat. Add the spinach and cook it until it's just wilted, about 1 to 2 minutes. Set aside.

Heat the remaining oil over medium heat. Cook the tofu slices until they have browned on both sides, about 5 to 8 minutes.

Divide the spinach, and tofu onto plates and drizzle the remaining yogurt sauce over the top.

Notes

- *Storage (for leftovers or meal prep):* Refrigerate in an airtight container for up to 2 days.
- *Serving size:* One serving equals approximately 1 cup rice, 4 ounces of tofu, and ½ cup spinach.
- *Add flavor:* Let the tofu marinate overnight. Add lime juice before serving.
- *Serving suggestion:* Serve with jasmice or brown rice.
- *Suggested additional toppings:* Add sliced green onions, parsley, or shredded coconut.

○ ○ ◉ ○ ○

AFTERWORD

In this book I have addressed the time-honored and up-to-date medical literature that demonstrates how very common leaky gut and dysbiosis are. Moreover, there is a critical link between a healthy digestive system, especially the small intestine and microbiome, and one's overall health. You now understand the importance of fostering healthy digestion for a high-quality and long life.

I highly recommend you take action to create a healthy gut. The foundation of great gut health is a consistently healthy diet. If your diet has not been healthy, then focus on the foods I have discussed that promote gut healing and restrict or reduce those foods that damage the gut. Moreover, incorporate the additional lifestyle factors that influence gut and body health, such as stress reduction, good sleep, detoxification, and exercise.

The body and digestive system have regenerative capacities that the methods I have discussed in this book tap into. If you provide the right environment through these holistic methods, then digestive healing will often occur. In addition, consultation with a holistic doctor or nutrition-oriented practitioner can help you identify specific areas of imbalance where you need help.

If you would like to stay up-to-date on holistic gut and whole-body health research and protocols, then sign up for my regular newsletter at www.markstengler.com.

I wish you all the best in your quest for optimal digestive and holistic health.

ENDNOTES

Introduction

1. "Physical Activity Helps Prevent Chronic Diseases," *Centers for Disease Control and Prevention*, May 8, 2023, https://www.cdc.gov/chronicdisease/index.htm.

Chapter 1

1. Siddhartha S. Ghosh et al., "Intestinal Barrier Dysfunction, LPS Translocation, and Disease Development," *Journal of the Endocrine Society* 4, no. 2 (February 1, 2020), https://doi.org/10.1210/jendso/bvz039.

2. Marcelo Campos, M.D. "Leaky Gut: What Is It, and What Does It Mean for You?" *Harvard Health Blog*, last modified November 16, 2021, https://www.health.harvard.edu/blog/leaky-gut-what-is-it-and-what-does-it-mean-for-you-2017092212451.

3. "Putting a Stop to Leaky Gut," *Harvard Health Publishing*, last modified December 1, 2018, https://www.health.harvard.edu/diseases-and-conditions/leaky-gut-putting-a-stop-to-this-mysterious-ailment.

4. Yusuke Kinashi and Koji Hase, "Partners in Leaky Gut Syndrome: Intestinal Dysbiosis and Autoimmunity," *Frontiers in Immunology* 12 (April 22, 2021), https://doi.org/10.3389/fimmu.2021.673708.

5. Alessio Fasano, "All Disease Begins in the (Leaky) Gut: Role of Zonulin-Mediated Gut Permeability in the Pathogenesis of Some Chronic Inflammatory Diseases," *F1000Research* 9 (January 31, 2020): 69, https://doi.org/10.12688/f1000research.20510.1.

6. Cezmi A. Akdis, "Does the Epithelial Barrier Hypothesis Explain the Increase in Allergy, Autoimmunity and Other Chronic Conditions?" *Nature Reviews Immunology* 21, no. 11 (November 12, 2021): 739–51, https://doi.org/10.1038/s41577-021-00538-7.

7. Herbert F. Helander and Lars Fändriks, "Surface Area of the Digestive Tract – Revisited," *Scandinavian Journal of Gastroenterology* 49, no. 6 (January 2, 2014): 681–89, https://doi.org/10.3109/00365521.2014.898326.

8. Ana G. Abril et al., "The Role of the Gallbladder, the Intestinal Barrier and the Gut Microbiota in the Development of Food Allergies and Other Disorders," *International Journal of Molecular Sciences* 23, no. 22 (November 18, 2022): 14333, https://doi.org/10.3390/ijms232214333.

9. Ibid.

10. Seun Ja Park, "Physiological Function of the Small Intestine," in *Small Intestine Disease: A Comprehensive Guide to Diagnosis and Management*, 7–11 (Singapore: Springer Verlag, 2022).

11. Elizabeth M. Fish and Bracken Burns, "Physiology, Small Bowel" in StatPearls NCBI Bookshelf (Treasure Island, FL: StatPearls Publishing; 2023 Jan).

12. Siddhartha S. Ghosh et al., "Intestinal Barrier Dysfunction, LPS Translocation, and Disease Development," *Journal of the Endocrine Society* 4, no. 2 (February 1, 2020), https://doi.org/10.1210/jendso/bvz039.

13. Sudha B. Singh and Henry C. Lin, "Role of Intestinal Alkaline Phosphatase in Innate Immunity." *Biomolecules* 11, no. 12 (November 29, 2021): 1784, https://doi.org/10.3390/biom11121784.

14. Tim Vanuytsel, Jan Tack, and Ricard Farre, "The Role of Intestinal Permeability in Gastrointestinal Disorders and Current Methods of Evaluation," *Frontiers in Nutrition* 8 (August 26, 2021), https://doi.org/10.3389/fnut.2021.717925.

15. Wenuki Song et al., "Identification and Structure–Activity Relationship of Intestinal Epithelial Barrier Function Protective Collagen Peptides from Alaska Pollock Skin," *Marine Drugs* 17, no. 8 (July 31, 2019): 450, https://doi.org/10.3390/md17080450.

16. Alessio Fasano, "Zonulin and Its Regulation of Intestinal Barrier Function: The Biological Door to Inflammation, Autoimmunity, and Cancer," *Physiological Reviews* 91, no. 1 (2011): 151–75, https://doi.org/10.1152/physrev.00003.2008.

17. Tim Vanuytsel, Jan Tack, and Ricard Farre, "The Role of Intestinal Permeability in Gastrointestinal Disorders and Current Methods of Evaluation," *Frontiers in Nutrition* 8 (August 26, 2021), https://doi.org/10.3389/fnut.2021.717925.

18. Xianglin Mei, Ming Gu, and Meiying Li, "Plasticity of Paneth Cells and Their Ability to Regulate Intestinal Stem Cells," *Stem Cell Research & Therapy* 11, no. 1 (August 12, 2020), https://doi.org/10.1186/s13287-020-01857-7.

19. William D. Rees et al., "Regenerative Intestinal Stem Cells Induced by Acute and Chronic Injury: The Saving Grace of the Epithelium?" *Frontiers in Cell and Developmental Biology* 8 (November 12, 2020), https://doi.org/10.3389/fcell.2020.583919.

20. Siddhartha S. Ghosh, Jing Wang, Paul J. Yannie, and Shobha Ghosh, "Intestinal Barrier Dysfunction, LPS Translocation, and Disease Development," *Journal of the Endocrine Society* 4, no. 2 (February 1, 2020), https://doi.org/10.1210/jendso/bvz039.

21. Ibid.

22. Ibid.

23. Ana G. Abril et al., "The Role of the Gallbladder, the Intestinal Barrier and the Gut Microbiota in the Development of Food Allergies and Other Disorders," *International Journal of Molecular Sciences* 23, no. 22 (November 18, 2022): 14333, https://doi.org/10.3390/ijms232214333.

24. Ibid.

25. Ronald Hills et al., "Gut Microbiome: Profound Implications for Diet and Disease," *Nutrients* 11, no. 7 (July 16, 2019): 1613, https://doi.org/10.3390/nu11071613.

26. Purna C. Kashyap et al., "Microbiome at the Frontier of Personalized Medicine," *Mayo Clinic Proceedings* 92, no. 12 (December 1, 2017): 1855–64, https://doi.org/10.1016/j.mayocp.2017.10.004.

27. Megan Clapp et al., "Gut Microbiota's Effect on Mental Health: The Gut-Brain Axis," *Clinics and Practice* 7, no. 4 (September 15, 2017): 987, https://doi.org/10.4081/cp.2017.987.

28. Jaime Ramirez et al., "Antibiotics as Major Disruptors of Gut Microbiota," *Frontiers in Cellular and Infection Microbiology* 10 (November 24, 2020), https://doi.org/10.3389/fcimb.2020.572912.

29. Christopher Staley, Thomas Kaiser, and Alexander Khoruts, "Clinician Guide to Microbiome Testing," *Digestive Diseases and Sciences* 63, no. 12 (2018): 3167–77, https://doi.org/10.1007/s10620-018-5299-6.

30. Rajan Singh et al., "Gut Microbial Dysbiosis in the Pathogenesis of Gastrointestinal Dysmotility and Metabolic Disorders," *Journal of Neurogastroenterology and Motility* 27, no. 1 (2021): 19–34, https://doi.org/10.5056/jnm20149.

31. Megan Clapp et al., "Gut Microbiota's Effect on Mental Health: The Gut-Brain Axis," *Clinics and Practice* 7, no. 4 (September 15, 2017), https://doi.org/10.4081/cp.2017.987.

32. Fergus Shanahan, Tarini S. Ghosh, and Paul W. O'Toole, "The Healthy Microbiome—What Is the Definition of a Healthy Gut Microbiome?" *Gastroenterology* 160, no. 2 (January 2021): 483–94, https://doi.org/10.1053/j.gastro.2020.09.057.

33. Tarini S. Ghosh et al., "Adjusting for Age Improves Identification of Gut Microbiome Alterations in Multiple Diseases," *eLife* 9 (March 11, 2020): e50240, https://doi.org/10.7554/elife.50240.

34. Arup Choudhury et al., "Gastrointestinal Manifestations of Long Covid: A Systematic Review and Meta-Analysis," *Therapeutic Advances in Gastroenterology* 15 (August 22, 2022): 175628482211184, https://doi.org/10.1177/17562848221118403.

Chapter 2

1. Bilal Ahmad Paray et al., "Leaky Gut and Autoimmunity: An Intricate Balance in Individuals Health and the Diseased State," *International Journal of Molecular Sciences* 21, no. 24 (December 21, 2020): 9770, https://doi.org/10.3390/ijms21249770.

2. Greta M. de Waal, Willem J. S. de Villiers, and Etheresia Pretorius, "The Link between Bacterial Inflammagens, Leaky Gut Syndrome and Colorectal Cancer," *Current Medicinal Chemistry* 28, no. 41 (February 19, 2021): 8534–48, https://doi.org/10.2174/0929867328666210219142737.

3. Greta M. de Waal et al., "Colorectal Cancer Is Associated with Increased Circulating Lipopolysaccharide, Inflammation and Hypercoagulability," *Scientific Reports* 10, no. 1 (May 29, 2020), https://doi.org/10.1038/s41598-020-65324-2.

4.   Allyson L. Byrd, Yasmine Belkaid, and Julia A. Segre, "The Human Skin Microbiome," *Nature Reviews Microbiology* 16, no. 3 (January 15, 2018): 143–55, https://doi.org/10.1038/nrmicro.2017.157.

5.   Priya Nimish Deo and Revati Deshmukh, "Oral Microbiome: Unveiling the Fundamentals," *Journal of Oral and Maxillofacial Pathology* 23, no. 1 (January 2019): 122–28, https://doi.org/10.4103/jomfp.jomfp_304_18.

6.   Laodong Li et al., "Probiotics for Preventing Upper Respiratory Tract Infections in Adults: A Systematic Review and Meta-Analysis of Randomized Controlled Trials," *Evidence-Based Complementary and Alternative Medicine* 2020 (October 26, 2020): 1–8. https://doi.org/10.1155/2020/8734140.

7.   I. La Mantia et al., "Probiotics in the Add-on Treatment of Pharyngotonsillitis: A Clinical Experience," *Journal of Biological Regulators and Homeostatic Agents* 34, no. 6 (n.d.): 11–18.

8.   Roopa Hebbandi Nanjundappa, Channakeshava Sokke Umeshappa, and Markus B. Geuking, "The Impact of the Gut Microbiota on T Cell Ontogeny in the Thymus," *Cellular and Molecular Life Sciences* 79, no. 4 (March 10, 2022), https://doi.org/10.1007/s00018-022-04252-y.

9.   Ibid.

10. Dachuan Zhang et al., "The Microbiota Regulates Hematopoietic Stem Cell Fate Decisions by Controlling Iron Availability in Bone Marrow," *Cell Stem Cell* 29, no. 2 (January 21, 2022), https://doi.org/10.1016/j.stem.2021.12.009.

11. I. A. Kooij et al., "The Immunology of the Vermiform Appendix: A Review of the Literature," *Clinical and Experimental Immunology* 186, no. 1 (July 19, 2016): 1–9, https://doi.org/10.1111/cei.12821.

12. Urs M. Mörbe et al., "Human Gut-Associated Lymphoid Tissues (Galt); Diversity, Structure, and Function," *Mucosal Immunology* 14, no. 4 (July 2021): 793–802, https://doi.org/10.1038/s41385-021-00389-4.

13. Alyce M. Martin et al., "The Influence of the Gut Microbiome on Host Metabolism through the Regulation of Gut Hormone Release," *Frontiers in Physiology* 10 (April 16, 2019), https://doi.org/10.3389/fphys.2019.00428.

14. Margarita Aguilera, Yolanda Gálvez-Ontiveros, and Ana Rivas, "Endobolome, a New Concept for Determining the Influence of Microbiota Disrupting Chemicals (MDC) in Relation to Specific Endocrine Pathogenesis," *Frontiers in Microbiology* 11 (November 30, 2020), https://doi.org/10.3389/fmicb.2020.578007.

15. Ibid.

16. Song He et al., "The Gut Microbiome and Sex Hormone-Related Diseases," *Frontiers in Microbiology* 12 (September 28, 2021), https://doi.org/10.3389/fmicb.2021.711137.

17. Albert Shieh et al., "Gut Permeability, Inflammation, and Bone Density across the Menopause Transition," *JCI Insight* 5, no. 2 (December 12, 2019), https://doi.org/10.1172/jci.insight.134092.

18. Samantha M. Ervin et al., "Gut Microbial [beta]-Glucuronidases Reactivate Estrogens as Components of the Estrobolome That Reactivate Estrogens,"

Journal of Biological Chemistry 294, no. 49 (October 21, 2019): 18586–99, https://doi.org/10.1074/jbc.ra119.010950.

19. Leonardo César Cayres et al., "Detection of Alterations in the Gut Micro-biota and Intestinal Permeability in Patients with Hashimoto Thyroiditis." *Frontiers in Immunology* 12 (March 5, 2021), https://doi.org/10.3389/fimmu.2021.579140.

20. Mara Ioana Iesanu et al., "Melatonin–Microbiome Two-Sided Interaction in Dysbiosis-Associated Conditions," *Antioxidants* 11, no. 11 (November 14, 2022): 2244, https://doi.org/10.3390/antiox11112244.

21. A. J. Cox et al., "Increased Intestinal Permeability as a Risk Factor for Type 2 Diabetes," *Diabetes & Metabolism* 43, no. 2 (April 2017): 163–66, https://doi.org/10.1016/j.diabet.2016.09.004.

22. Lili Zhang et al., "Gut Microbiota and Type 2 Diabetes Mellitus: Association, Mechanism, and Translational Applications," *Mediators of Inflammation* 2021 (August 17, 2021): 1–12, https://doi.org/10.1155/2021/5110276.

23. Lulu Liu et al., "Gut Microbiota: A New Target for T2DM Prevention and Treatment," *Frontiers in Endocrinology* 13 (August 11, 2022), https://doi.org/10.3389/fendo.2022.958218.

24. Ibid.

25. Alyce M. Martin et al., "The Influence of the Gut Microbiome on Host Metabolism through the Regulation of Gut Hormone Release," *Frontiers in Physiology* 10 (April 16, 2019), https://doi.org/10.3389/fphys.2019.00428.

26. Laila Al-Ayadhi et al., "The Use of Biomarkers Associated with Leaky Gut as a Diagnostic Tool for Early Intervention in Autism Spectrum Disorder: A Systematic Review," *Gut Pathogens* 13, no. 1 (August 13, 2021), https://doi.org/10.1186/s13099-021-00448-y.

27. Mark Obrenovich, "Leaky Gut, Leaky Brain?" *Microorganisms* 6, no. 4 (October 18, 2018): 107, https://doi.org/10.3390/microorganisms6040107.

28. Ibid.

29. Ibid.

30. Brett J. Deters and Mir Saleem. "The Role of Glutamine in Supporting Gut Health and Neuropsychiatric Factors," *Food Science and Human Wellness* 10, no. 2 (March 2021): 149–54, https://doi.org/10.1016/j.fshw.2021.02.003.

31. Annelise Madison and Janice K Kiecolt-Glaser, "Stress, Depression, Diet, and the Gut Microbiota: Human–Bacteria Interactions at the Core of Psychoneuroimmunology and Nutrition," *Current Opinion in Behavioral Sciences* 28 (March 15, 2019): 105–10, https://doi.org/10.1016/j.cobeha.2019.01.011.

32. Jenelle Marcelle Safadi et al., "Gut Dysbiosis in Severe Mental Illness and Chronic Fatigue: A Novel Trans-Diagnostic Construct? A Systematic Review and Meta-Analysis," *Molecular Psychiatry* 27, no. 1 (January 8, 2021): 141–53, https://doi.org/10.1038/s41380-021-01032-1.

33. Veena Taneja, "Arthritis Susceptibility and the Gut Microbiome," *FEBS Letters* 588, no. 22 (November 27, 2014): 4244–49, https://doi.org/10.1016/j.febslet.2014.05.034.

34. Yusuke Kinashi and Koji Hase, "Partners in Leaky Gut Syndrome: Intestinal Dysbiosis and Autoimmunity," *Frontiers in Immunology* 12 (April 22, 2021), https://doi.org/10.3389/fimmu.2021.673708.

35. Deena Dahshan et al., "Targeting the Gut Microbiome for Inflammation and Pain Management in Orthopedic Conditions," *Orthopedics* 45, no. 5 (June 2022), https://doi.org/10.3928/01477447-20220608-07.

36. Ye Tu et al., "The Microbiota-Gut-Bone Axis and Bone Health." *Journal of Leukocyte Biology* 110, no. 3 (April 22, 2021): 525–37, https://doi.org/10.1002/jlb.3mr0321-755r.

37. Albert Shieh et al., "Gut Permeability, Inflammation, and Bone Density across the Menopause Transition," *JCI Insight* 5, no. 2 (December 12, 2019), https://doi.org/10.1172/jci.insight.134092.

38. A. G. Nilsson et al., "Lactobacillus Reuteri Reduces Bone Loss in Older Women with Low Bone Mineral Density: A Randomized, Placebo-Controlled, Double-Blind, Clinical Trial," *Journal of Internal Medicine* 284, no. 3 (2018): 307–317, https://doi.org/10.1111/joim.12805.

39. Esther Forkosh and Yaron Ilan, "The Heart-Gut Axis: New Target for Atherosclerosis and Congestive Heart Failure Therapy," *Open Heart* 6, no. 1 (April 23, 2019), https://doi.org/10.1136/openhrt-2018-000993.

40. Marko Novakovic et al., "Role of Gut Microbiota in Cardiovascular Diseases," *World Journal of Cardiology* 12, no. 4 (April 26, 2020): 110–22, https://doi.org/10.4330/wjc.v12.i4.110.

41. Allison Clark and Núria Mach, "The Crosstalk between the Gut Microbiota and Mitochondria during Exercise," *Frontiers in Physiology* 8 (May 19, 2017), https://doi.org/10.3389/fphys.2017.00319.

42. Jenelle Marcelle Safadi et al., "Gut Dysbiosis in Severe Mental Illness and Chronic Fatigue: A Novel Trans-Diagnostic Construct? A Systematic Review and Meta-Analysis," *Molecular Psychiatry* 27, no. 1 (January 8, 2021): 141–53, https://doi.org/10.1038/s41380-021-01032-1.

43. Meštrovic, Tomislav et al., "The Role of Gut, Vaginal, and Urinary Microbiome in Urinary Tract Infections: From Bench to Bedside," *Diagnostics* 11, no. 1 (December 22, 2020): 7, https://doi.org/10.3390/diagnostics11010007.

44. Kevin M. Byrd and Ajay S. Gulati, "The 'Gum–Gut' Axis in Inflammatory Bowel Diseases: A Hypothesis-Driven Review of Associations and Advances," *Frontiers in Immunology* 12 (February 19, 2021), https://doi.org/10.3389/fimmu.2021.620124.

45. Ingar Olsen and Kazuhisa Yamazaki, "Can Oral Bacteria Affect the Microbiome of the Gut?" *Journal of Oral Microbiology* 11, no. 1 (March 18, 2019): 1586422, https://doi.org/10.1080/20002297.2019.1586422.

46. Pasquale Napolitano et al., "Influence of Gut Microbiota on Eye Diseases: An Overview," *Annals of Medicine* 53, no. 1 (May 1, 2021): 750–61, https://doi.org/10.1080/07853890.2021.1925150.

47. Gianluca Scuderi, Emidio Troiani, and Angelo Maria Minnella, "Gut Microbiome in Retina Health: The Crucial Role of the Gut-Retina Axis," *Frontiers in Microbiology* 12 (January 14, 2022), https://doi.org/10.3389/fmicb.2021.726792.

48. Xiaodi Chen, Yune Lu, Tao Chen, and Rongguo Li, "The Female Vaginal Microbiome in Health and Bacterial Vaginosis," *Frontiers in Cellular and Infection Microbiology* 11 (April 7, 2021), https://doi.org/10.3389/fcimb.2021.631972.

49. Emmanuel Amabebe and Dilly O. Anumba, "Female Gut and Genital Tract Microbiota-Induced Crosstalk and Differential Effects of Short-Chain Fatty Acids on Immune Sequelae," *Frontiers in Immunology* 11 (September 10, 2020), https://doi.org/10.3389/fimmu.2020.02184.

50. Yan Wang and Zuogang Xie, "Exploring the Role of Gut Microbiome in Male Reproduction," *Andrology* 10, no. 3 (September 5, 2022): 441–50, https://doi.org/10.1111/andr.13143.

51. Bijan Helli et al., "Probiotic Effects on Sperm Parameters, Oxidative Stress Index, Inflammatory Factors and Sex Hormones in Infertile Men," *Human Fertility* 25, no. 3 (September 27, 2020): 499–507, https://doi.org/10.1080/14647273.2020.1824080.

52. E. A. Mann et al., "The Gut Microbiome: Human Health and Inflammatory Skin Diseases," *Annals of Dermatology* 32, no. 4 (June 30, 2020): 265–272, https://doi.org/10.5021/ad.2020.32.4.265.

53. Ibid.

54. I. Hamilton et al., "Small Intestinal Permeability in Dermatological Disease," *The Quarterly Journal of Medicine* 56, no. 221 (1985): 559–567.

55. Sandrine P. Claus, Hervé Guillou, and Sandrine Ellero-Simatos, "The Gut Microbiota: A Major Player in the Toxicity of Environmental Pollutants?" *npj Biofilms and Microbiomes* 2, no. 1 (May 4, 2016), https://doi.org/10.1038/npjbiofilms.2016.3.

56. Stephanie L. Collins and Andrew D. Patterson, "The Gut Microbiome: An Orchestrator of Xenobiotic Metabolism," *Acta Pharmaceutica Sinica B* 10, no. 1 (December 10, 2019): 19–32, https://doi.org/10.1016/j.apsb.2019.12.001.

57. Priyanka Bist and Sangeeta Choudhary, "Impact of Heavy Metal Toxicity on the Gut Microbiota and Its Relationship with Metabolites and Future Probiotics Strategy: A Review," *Biological Trace Element Research* 200, no. 12 (January 7, 2022): 5328–50, https://doi.org/10.1007/s12011-021-03092-4.

58. Alexander C. Ford, Ami D. Sperber, Maura Corsetti, and Michael Camilleri, "Irritable Bowel Syndrome," *The Lancet* 396, no. 10263 (October 10, 2020): 1675–88, https://doi.org/10.1016/s0140-6736(20)31548-8.

59. Bilal Ahmad Paray, Mohammed Fahad Albeshr, Arif Tasleem Jan, and Irfan A. Rather, "Leaky Gut and Autoimmunity: An Intricate Balance in Individuals

Health and the Diseased State," *International Journal of Molecular Sciences* 21, no. 24 (December 21, 2020): 9770; Alexander C. Ford et al., "Irritable Bowel Syndrome," *The Lancet* 396, no. 10263 (October 10, 2020): 1675–88, https://doi.org/10.1016/s0140-6736(20)31548-8.

Chapter 3

1. Ravinder Nagpal et al., "Gut Microbiome and Aging: Physiological and Mechanistic Insights," *Nutrition and Healthy Aging* 4, no. 4 (June 15, 2018): 267–85, https://doi.org/10.3233/nha-170030.

2. Nabil Bosco and Mario Noti, "The Aging Gut Microbiome and Its Impact on Host Immunity," *Genes & Immunity* 22, no. 5–6 (April 19, 2021): 289–303, https://doi.org/10.1038/s41435-021-00126-8.

3. Faraz Bishehsari et al., "Alcohol and Gut-Derived Inflammation," *Alcohol Research* 38, no. 2 (2017): 163–71.

4. Ann Cecile Muls, "Gastrointestinal Consequences of Cancer Treatment and the Wider Context: A Bad Gut Feeling," *Acta Oncologica* 53, no. 3 (January 27, 2014): 297–306, https://doi.org/10.3109/0284186x.2013.873140.

5. Juliana E. Bajic et al., "From the Bottom-up: Chemotherapy and Gut-Brain Axis Dysregulation," *Frontiers in Behavioral Neuroscience* 12 (May 22, 2018), https://doi.org/10.3389/fnbeh.2018.00104.

6. Tomoko Kumagai, Farooq Rahman, and Andrew Smith, "The Microbiome and Radiation Induced-Bowel Injury: Evidence for Potential Mechanistic Role in Disease Pathogenesis," *Nutrients* 10, no. 10 (October 2, 2018): 1405, https://doi.org/10.3390/nu10101405.

7. Jing Liu, Chao Liu, and Jinbo Yue, "Radiotherapy and the Gut Microbiome: Facts and Fiction," *Radiation Oncology* 16, no. 1 (January 13, 2021), https://doi.org/10.1186/s13014-020-01735-9.

8. Meng-Meng Liu et al., "Probiotics for Prevention of Radiation-Induced Diarrhea: A Meta-Analysis of Randomized Controlled Trials," *PLOS ONE* 12, no. 6 (June 2, 2017), https://doi.org/10.1371/journal.pone.0178870.

9. K. C. Konturek, T. Brzozowski, and S. J. Konturek, "Stress and the Gut: Pathophysiology, Clinical Consequences, Diagnostic Approach and Treatment Options," *Journal of Physiology and Pharmacology* 62, no. 6 (2011).

10. Meri K. Tulic et al., "Presence of Commensal House Dust Mite Allergen in Human Gastrointestinal Tract: A Potential Contributor to Intestinal Barrier Dysfunction," *Gut* 65 (2016): 757–66, https://doi.org/10.1136/gutjnl-2015-310523.

11. Yusuke Kinashi and Koji Hase, "Partners in Leaky Gut Syndrome: Intestinal Dysbiosis and Autoimmunity," *Frontiers in Immunology* 12 (April 22, 2021), https://doi.org/10.3389/fimmu.2021.673708.

12. Filipe M. Ribeiro et al., "Is There an Exercise-Intensity Threshold Capable of Avoiding the Leaky Gut?" *Frontiers in Nutrition* 8 (March 8, 2021), https://doi.org/10.3389/fnut.2021.627289.

13. Ibid.

14. S. Buhner, et al., "Genetic Basis for Increased Intestinal Permeability in Families with Crohn's Disease: Role of Card15 3020INSC Mutation?" *Gut* 55, no. 3 (March 1, 2006): 342–47, https://doi.org/10.1136/gut.2005.065557.

15. M. C. Lomer, "Review Article: The Aetiology, Diagnosis, Mechanisms and Clinical Evidence for Food Intolerance," *Alimentary Pharmacology & Therapeutics* 41, no. 3 (December 3, 2014): 262–75, https://doi.org/10.1111/apt.13041.

16. Aitak Farzi, Esther E. Fröhlich, and Peter Holzer, "Gut Microbiota and the Neuroendocrine System," *Neurotherapeutics* 15, no. 1 (January 15, 2018): 5–22, https://doi.org/10.1007/s13311-017-0600-5.

17. Laila Al-Ayadhi et al., "The Use of Biomarkers Associated with Leaky Gut as a Diagnostic Tool for Early Intervention in Autism Spectrum Disorder: A Systematic Review," *Gut Pathogens* 13, no. 1 (September 13, 2021), https://doi.org/10.1186/s13099-021-00448-y.

18. Lei Yan, Chunhui Yang, and Jianguo Tang, "Disruption of the Intestinal Mucosal Barrier in Candida Albicans Infections," *Microbiological Research* 168, no. 7 (August 25, 2013): 389–95, https://doi.org/10.1016/j.micres.2013.02.008.

19. Ibid.

20. "Parasites - Neglected Parasitic Infections (Npis) in the United States," *Centers for Disease Control*, November 20, 2020, https://www.cdc.gov/parasites/npi/index.html.

21. Peijie Zhong et al., "Covid-19-Associated Gastrointestinal and Liver Injury: Clinical Features and Potential Mechanisms," *Signal Transduction and Targeted Therapy* 5, no. 1 (November 2, 2020), https://doi.org/10.1038/s41392-020-00373-7.

22. Damian Maseda and Emanuela Ricciotti, "NSAID–Gut Microbiota Interactions," *Frontiers in Pharmacology* 11 (August 7, 2020), https://doi.org/10.3389/fphar.2020.01153.

23. "Nearly 7 in 10 Americans Take Prescription Drugs, Mayo Clinic, Olmsted Medical Center Find," *Mayo Clinic*, June 19, 2013. https://newsnetwork.mayoclinic.org/discussion/nearly-7-in-10-americans-take-prescription-drugs-mayo-clinic-olmsted-medical-center-find.

24. Lisa Maier et al., "Extensive Impact of Non-Antibiotic Drugs on Human Gut Bacteria," *Nature* 555, no. 7698 (March 19, 2018): 623–28, https://doi.org/10.1038/nature25979.

25. Damian Maseda and Emanuela Ricciotti, "NSAID–Gut Microbiota Interactions." *Frontiers in Pharmacology* 11 (August 7, 2020), https://doi.org/10.3389/fphar.2020.01153.

26. H. Gelberg, "Pathophysiological Mechanisms of Gastrointestinal Toxicity," *Comprehensive Toxicology* (November 27, 2017): 139–78, https://doi.org/10.1016/b978-0-12-801238-3.10923-7.

27. Damian Maseda and Emanuela Ricciotti, "NSAID–Gut Microbiota Interactions." *Frontiers in Pharmacology* 11 (August 7, 2020), https://doi .org/10.3389/fphar.2020.01153.

28. Mi Young Yoon and Sang Sun Yoon, "Disruption of the Gut Ecosystem by Antibiotics," *Yonsei Medical Journal* 59, no. 1 (January 2018): 4, https://doi .org/10.3349/ymj.2018.59.1.4.

29. Jinqiu Yuan et al., "Long-Term Use of Antibiotics and Risk of Type 2 Diabetes in Women: A Prospective Cohort Study," *International Journal of Epidemiology* 49, no. 5 (September 7, 2020): 1572–81, https://doi.org/10.1093/ije/dyaa122.

30. Thomas G. Cotter and Mary Rinella, "Nonalcoholic Fatty Liver Disease 2020: The State of the Disease," *Gastroenterology* 158, no. 7 (2020): 1851–64, https://doi.org/10.1053/j.gastro.2020.01.052.

31. Takaomi Kessoku et al., "The Role of Leaky Gut in Nonalcoholic Fatty Liver Disease: A Novel Therapeutic Target," *International Journal of Molecular Sciences* 22, no. 15 (July 29, 2021): 8161, https://doi.org /10.3390/ijms22158161.

32. Sergio Quesada-Vázquez et al., "Microbiota Dysbiosis and Gut Barrier Dysfunction Associated with Non-Alcoholic Fatty Liver Disease Are Modulated by a Specific Metabolic Cofactors' Combination," *International Journal of Molecular Sciences* 23, no. 22 (November 8, 2022): 13675, https:// doi.org/10.3390/ijms232213675.

33. Ricard Farré et al., "Intestinal Permeability, Inflammation and the Role of Nutrients," *Nutrients* 12, no. 4 (April 23, 2020): 1185, https://doi.org /10.3390/nu12041185.

34. Emidio Scarpellini et al., "Zinc and Gut Microbiota in Health and Gastrointestinal Disease under the COVID-19 Suggestion," *BioFactors* 48, no. 2 (February 26, 2022): 294–306, https://doi.org/10.1002/biof.1829.

35. Lara Costantini et al., "Impact of Omega-3 Fatty Acids on the Gut Microbiota," *International Journal of Molecular Sciences* 18, no. 12 (December 7, 2017): 2645, https://doi.org/10.3390/ijms18122645.
    Luke A. Durkin, Caroline E. Childs, and Philip C. Calder, "Omega-3 Polyunsaturated Fatty Acids and the Intestinal Epithelium—a Review," *Foods* 10, no. 1 (January 19, 2021): 199, https://doi.org/10.3390/foods10010199.

36. Katayoun Khoshbin and Michael Camilleri, "Effects of Dietary Components on Intestinal Permeability in Health and Disease," *American Journal of Physiology: Neurogastroenterology and Motility* 319, no. 5 (November 3, 2020), https://doi.org/10.1152/ajpgi.00245.2020.

37. Juliana E. Bajic et al., "From the Bottom-up: Chemotherapy and Gut-Brain Axis Dysregulation," *Frontiers in Behavioral Neuroscience* 12 (May 22, 2018), https://doi.org/10.3389/fnbeh.2018.00104.

38. Annelise Madison and Janice K Kiecolt-Glaser, "Stress, Depression, Diet, and the Gut Microbiota: Human–Bacteria Interactions at the Core of Psychoneuroimmunology and Nutrition," *Current Opinion in Behavioral Sciences* 28 (March 25, 2019): 105–10, https://doi.org/10.1016 /j.cobeha.2019.01.011.

39. Jason E. Martinez et al., "Unhealthy Lifestyle and Gut Dysbiosis: A Better Understanding of the Effects of Poor Diet and Nicotine on the Intestinal Microbiome," *Frontiers in Endocrinology* 12 (June 8, 2021), https://doi.org /10.3389/fendo.2021.667066.

40. Loni Berkowitz et al., "Impact of Cigarette Smoking on the Gastrointestinal Tract Inflammation: Opposing Effects in Crohn's Disease and Ulcerative Colitis," *Frontiers in Immunology* 9, no. 74 (January 30, 2018), https://doi .org/10.3389/fimmu.2018.00074.

41. "Obesity and Overweight," *Centers for Disease Control and Prevention*, September 6, 2022, https://www.cdc.gov/nchs/fastats/obesity -overweight.htm.

42. Antje Damms-Machado et al., "Gut Permeability Is Related to Body Weight, Fatty Liver Disease, and Insulin Resistance in Obese Individuals Undergoing Weight Reduction," *The American Journal of Clinical Nutrition* 105, no. 1 (January 2017): 127–35, https://doi.org/10.3945/ajcn.116.131110.

43. M. J. Saad, A. Santos, and P. O. Prada, "Linking Gut Microbiota and Inflammation to Obesity and Insulin Resistance," *Physiology* 31, no. 4 (June 2016): 283–93, https://doi.org/10.1152/physiol.00041.2015.

44. Ibid.

45. Lusikelelwe Mkumbuzi et al., "Insulin Resistance Is Associated with Gut Permeability without the Direct Influence of Obesity in Young Adults," *Diabetes, Metabolic Syndrome and Obesity: Targets and Therapy* Volume 13 (August 24, 2020): 2997–3008, https://doi.org/10.2147/dmso.s256864.

46. "An Estimated 12.6 Million Deaths Each Year Are Attributable to Unhealthy Environments," *World Health Organization*, March 15, 2016, https://www .who.int/news/item/15-03-2016-an-estimated-12-6-million-deaths-each -year-are-attributable-to-unhealthy-environments.

47. Firas Alhasson et al., "Altered Gut Microbiome in a Mouse Model of Gulf War Illness Causes Neuroinflammation and Intestinal Injury via Leaky Gut and TLR4 Activation," *PLOS ONE* 12, no. 3 (March 22, 2017), https://doi.org /10.1371/journal.pone.0172914.

48. Hoda Elkafas et al., "Gut and Genital Tract Microbiomes: Dysbiosis and Link to Gynecological Disorders," *Frontiers in Cellular and Infection Microbiology* 12 (December 16, 2022), https://doi.org/10.3389/fcimb.2022.1059825.

49. Pengcheng Tu et al., "Gut Microbiome Toxicity: Connecting the Environment and Gut Microbiome-Associated Diseases," *Toxics* 8, no. 1 (March 12, 2020): 19, https://doi.org/10.3390/toxics8010019.

50. Ibid.

51. Lola Rueda-Ruzafa et al., "Gut Microbiota and Neurological Effects of Glyphosate," *NeuroToxicology* 75 (December 2019): 1–8, https://doi.org /10.1016/j.neuro.2019.08.006.

52. Jacqueline A. Barnett and Deanna L. Gibson, "Separating the Empirical Wheat from the Pseudoscientific Chaff: A Critical Review of the Literature

Surrounding Glyphosate, Dysbiosis and Wheat-Sensitivity," *Frontiers in Microbiology* 11 (2020), https://doi.org/10.3389/fmicb.2020.556729.

53. Ibid.

54. Alessio Fasano, "All Disease Begins in the (Leaky) Gut: Role of Zonulin-Mediated Gut Permeability in the Pathogenesis of Some Chronic Inflammatory Diseases," *F1000Research* 9 (January 31, 2020): 69, https://doi.org/10.12688/f1000research.20510.1.

55. Laila Al-Ayadhi et al., "The Use of Biomarkers Associated with Leaky Gut as a Diagnostic Tool for Early Intervention in Autism Spectrum Disorder: A Systematic Review," *Gut Pathogens* 13, no. 1 (August 13, 2021), https://doi.org/10.1186/s13099-021-00448-y.

56. Md. Abu Musa et al., "Measurement of Intestinal Permeability Using Lactulose and Mannitol with Conventional Five Hours and Shortened Two Hours Urine Collection by Two Different Methods: HPAE-Pad and LC-MSMS," *PLOS ONE* 14, no. 8 (August 8, 2019), https://doi.org/10.1371/journal.pone.0220397.

57. Christopher Staley, Thomas Kaiser, and Alexander Khoruts, "Clinician Guide to Microbiome Testing," *Digestive Diseases and Sciences* 63, no. 12 (2018): 3167–77, https://doi.org/10.1007/s10620-018-5299-6.

Chapter 4

1. Catarina Sousa Guerreiro et al., "Diet, Microbiota, and Gut Permeability—the Unknown Triad in Rheumatoid Arthritis," *Frontiers in Medicine* 5 (December 14, 2018), https://doi.org/10.3389/fmed.2018.00349.

2. Laila Al-Ayadhi et al., "The Use of Biomarkers Associated with Leaky Gut as a Diagnostic Tool for Early Intervention in Autism Spectrum Disorder: A Systematic Review," *Gut Pathogens* 13, no. 1 (August 13, 2021), https://doi.org/10.1186/s13099-021-00448-y.

3. Ibid.

4. Carmen Haro et al., "Two Healthy Diets Modulate Gut Microbial Community Improving Insulin Sensitivity in a Human Obese Population," *The Journal of Clinical Endocrinology & Metabolism* 101, no. 1 (January 1, 2016): 233–42, https://doi.org/10.1210/jc.2015-3351.

5. Victoria Meslier et al., "Mediterranean Diet Intervention in Overweight and Obese Subjects Lowers Plasma Cholesterol and Causes Changes in the Gut Microbiome and Metabolome Independently of Energy Intake," *Gut* 69, no. 7 (July 19, 2020): 1258–68, https://doi.org/10.1136/gutjnl-2019-320438.

6. Tarini Shankar Ghosh et al., "Mediterranean Diet Intervention Alters the Gut Microbiome in Older People Reducing Frailty and Improving Health Status: The Nu-Age 1-Year Dietary Intervention across Five European Countries," *Gut* 69, no. 7 (February 17, 2020): 1218–28, https://doi.org/10.1136/gutjnl-2019-319654.

7. Dorna Davani-Davari et al., "Prebiotics: Definition, Types, Sources, Mechanisms, and Clinical Applications." *Foods* 8, no. 3 (March 9, 2019): 92, https://doi.org/10.3390/foods8030092.

8. Ibid.

9. Hannah Cory et al., "The Role of Polyphenols in Human Health and Food Systems: A Mini-Review," *Frontiers in Nutrition* 5 (September 21, 2018), https://doi.org/10.3389/fnut.2018.00087.

10. Ricardo Santos Aleman, Marvin Moncada, and Kayanush J. Aryana, "Leaky Gut and the Ingredients That Help Treat It: A Review." *Molecules* 28, no. 2 (January 7, 2023): 619, https://doi.org/10.3390/molecules28020619.

11. Diane Quagliani and Patricia Felt-Gunderson, "Closing America's Fiber Intake Gap," *American Journal of Lifestyle Medicine* 11, no. 1 (July 7, 2016): 80–85, https://doi.org/10.1177/1559827615588079.

12. Marcin Krawczyk et al., "Gut Permeability Might Be Improved by Dietary Fiber in Individuals with Nonalcoholic Fatty Liver Disease (NAFLD) Undergoing Weight Reduction," *Nutrients* 10, no. 11 (November 18, 2018): 1793, https://doi.org/10.3390/nu10111793.

13. Dorna Davani-Davari et al., "Prebiotics: Definition, Types, Sources, Mechanisms, and Clinical Applications," *Foods* 8, no. 3 (March 9, 2019): 92, https://doi.org/10.3390/foods8030092.

14. F. C. Ribeiro et al., "Action Mechanisms of Probiotics on *Candida* Spp. and Candidiasis Prevention: An Update," *Journal of Applied Microbiology* 129, no. 2 (November 21, 2019): 175–85, https://doi.org/10.1111/jam.14511.

15. "Probiotics: What You Need to Know," *National Center for Complementary and Integrative Health, U.S. Department of Health and Human Services*, last modified July 2019, https://www.nccih.nih.gov/health/probiotics-what-you-need-to-know.

16. "Probiotics," *International Scientific Association for Probiotics and Prebiotics (ISAPP)*, December 2, 2021, https://isappscience.org/for-scientists/resources/probiotics.

17. "Probiotics," *NIH Office of Dietary Supplements*, June 2, 2022, https://ods.od.nih.gov/factsheets/Probiotics-HealthProfessional.

18. Radha Krishna Rao and Geetha Samak, "Protection and Restitution of Gut Barrier by Probiotics: Nutritional and Clinical Implications," *Current Nutrition and Food Science* 9, no. 2 (May 1, 2013): 99–107, https://doi.org/10.2174/1573401311309020004.

19. Rout George Kerry et al., "Benefaction of Probiotics for Human Health: A Review," *Journal of Food and Drug Analysis* 26, no. 3 (July 2018): 927–39, https://doi.org/10.1016/j.jfda.2018.01.002.

20. "Probiotics," *NIH Office of Dietary Supplements*, June 2, 2022, https://ods.od.nih.gov/factsheets/Probiotics-HealthProfessional.

21. Yong Wen et al., "The Efficacy and Safety of Probiotics for Patients with Constipation-Predominant Irritable Bowel Syndrome: A Systematic Review

and Meta-Analysis Based on Seventeen Randomized Controlled Trials," *International Journal of Surgery* 79 (July 2020): 111–19, https://doi.org /10.1016/j.ijsu.2020.04.063.

22. Damini Kothari, Seema Patel, and Soo-Ki Kim, "Probiotic Supplements Might Not Be Universally-Effective and Safe: A Review," *Biomedicine & Pharmacotherapy* 111 (March 2019): 537–47, https://doi.org/10.1016 /j.biopha.2018.12.104.

23. Sameer Sharif et al., "Probiotics in Critical Illness: A Systematic Review and Meta-Analysis of Randomized Controlled Trials," *Critical Care Medicine* 50, no. 8 (August 25, 2022): 1175–86, https://doi.org/10.1097 /ccm.0000000000005580.

24. Valeria Agamennone et al., "A Practical Guide for Probiotics Applied to the Case of Antibiotic-Associated Diarrhea in the Netherlands," *BMC Gastroenterology* 18, no. 1 (August 6, 2018), https://doi.org/10.1186 /s12876-018-0831-x.

25. Jakub Zółkiewicz et al., "Postbiotics—a Step beyond Pre- and Probiotics," *Nutrients* 12, no. 8 (July 23, 2020): 2189, https://doi.org/10.3390/nu12082189.

26. Belinda Vallejo-Cordoba et al., Chapter 1 in *Probiotic and Prebiotics in Foods: Challenges, Innovations and Advances* 94 (Cambridge, MA: Academic Press, 2020), 1–34.

27. Rao Shripada, Athalye-Jape Gayatri, and Patole Sanjay, "Chapter 5-Paraprobiotics," in *Precision Medicine for Investigators, Practitioners and Providers* (Academic Press, 2020), 39–49.

28. L. Zorzela et al., "Is There a Role for Modified Probiotics as Beneficial Microbes: A Systematic Review of the Literature," *Beneficial Microbes* 8, no. 5 (October 13, 2017): 739–54, https://doi.org/10.3920/bm2017.0032.

29. Jakub Zółkiewicz et al.. "Postbiotics—a Step beyond Pre- and Probiotics," *Nutrients* 12, no. 8 (July 23, 2020): 2189, https://doi.org/10.3390 /nu12082189.

30. Lara Costantini et al., "Impact of Omega-3 Fatty Acids on the Gut Microbiota," *International Journal of Molecular Sciences* 18, no. 12 (December 7, 2017): 2645, https://doi.org/10.3390/ijms18122645.

31. Siddhartha S. Ghosh et al., "Curcumin-Mediated Regulation of Intestinal Barrier Function: The Mechanism Underlying Its Beneficial Effects," *Tissue Barriers* 6, no. 1 (February 2, 2018), https://doi.org/10.1080/21688370 .2018.1425085.

32. Natasha K. Leeuwendaal et al., "Fermented Foods, Health and the Gut Microbiome," *Nutrients* 14, no. 7 (April 6, 2022): 1527, https://doi.org /10.3390/nu14071527.

33. Ibid.

34. Leah T. Stiemsma et al., "Does Consumption of Fermented Foods Modify the Human Gut Microbiota?" *The Journal of Nutrition* 150, no. 7 (July 31, 2020): 1680–92, https://doi.org/10.1093/jn/nxaa077.

35. Robin Mesnage et al., "Changes in Human Gut Microbiota Composition Are Linked to the Energy Metabolic Switch during 10 D of Buchinger Fasting," *Journal of Nutritional Science* 8 (November 12, 2019), https://doi.org/10.1017/jns.2019.33.

36. Beate Ott et al, "Effect of Caloric Restriction on Gut Permeability, Inflammation Markers, and Fecal Microbiota in Obese Women," *Scientific Reports* 7, no. 1 (September 20, 2017), https://doi.org/10.1038/s41598-017-12109-9.

37. Guoxian Wei et al., "Gluten Degrading Enzymes for Treatment of Celiac Disease," *Nutrients* 12, no. 7 (July 15, 2020): 2095, https://doi.org/10.3390/nu12072095.

38. Samuel O. Igbinedion et al., "Non-Celiac Gluten Sensitivity: All Wheat Attack Is Not Celiac," *World Journal of Gastroenterology* 23, no. 40 (October 28, 2017): 7201–10, https://doi.org/10.3748/wjg.v23.i40.7201.

39. Moon Do et al., "High-Glucose or -Fructose Diet Cause Changes of the Gut Microbiota and Metabolic Disorders in Mice without Body Weight Change," *Nutrients* 10, no. 6 (June 13, 2018): 761, https://doi.org/10.3390/nu10060761.

40. Federica Laudisi, Carmine Stolfi, and Giovanni Monteleone, "Impact of Food Additives on Gut Homeostasis," *Nutrients* 11, no. 10 (October 1, 2019): 2334, https://doi.org/10.3390/nu11102334.

41. Abigail Raffner Basson, Alexander Rodriguez-Palacios, and Fabio Cominelli, "Artificial Sweeteners: History and New Concepts on Inflammation," *Frontiers in Nutrition* 8 (September 24, 2021), https://doi.org/10.3389/fnut.2021.746247.

42. Shao-Cheng Wang et al., "Alcohol Addiction, Gut Microbiota, and Alcoholism Treatment: A Review," *International Journal of Molecular Sciences* 21, no. 17 (September 3, 2020): 6413, https://doi.org/10.3390/ijms21176413.

43. Ibid.

44. Alexandra Adorno Vita, Heather Zwickey, and Ryan Bradley, "Associations between Food-Specific IGG Antibodies and Intestinal Permeability Biomarkers," *Frontiers in Nutrition* 9 (September 6, 2022), https://doi.org/10.3389/fnut.2022.962093.

Chapter 5

1. T. Prueksrisakul, S. Chantarangsu, and P. Thunyakitpisal, "Effect of Daily Drinking of Aloe Vera Gel Extract on Plasma Total Antioxidant Capacity and Oral Pathogenic Bacteria in Healthy Volunteer: A Short-term Study," *Journal of Complementary and Integrative Medicine* 12, no. 2 (2015): 159–164, https://doi.org/10.1515/jcim-2014-0060.

2. H. Lin et al., "The Mechanism of Alopolysaccharide Protecting Ulceralive Colitis," *Biomedicine & Pharmacotherapy* 88 (April 2017): 145–150, https://doi.org/10.1016/j.biopha.2016.11.138.

3. Le Phan et al., "The Role of Processed Aloe Vera Gel in Intestinal Tight Junction: An In vivo and In vitro Study," *International Journal of Molecular Sciences* 22, no. 12 (2021): 6515, https://doi.org/10.3390/ijms22126515.

4. Y. Panahi et al., "Efficacy and Safety of Aloe Vera Syrup for the Treatment of Gastroesophageal Reflux Disease: A Pilot Randomized Positive-controlled Trial," *Journal of Traditional Chinese Medicine* 35, no. 6 (December 2015): 632–636, https://doi.org/10.1016/s0254-6272(15)30151-5.

5. S. W. Hong et al., "Aloe Vera Is Effective and Safe In Short-Term Treatment of Irritable Bowel Syndrome: A Systematic Review and Meta-Analysis," *Journal of Neurogastroenterology and Motility* 24, no. 4 (2018): 528–535. https://doi.org/10.5056/jnm18077.

6. Giulia Pastorino et al., "Liquorice (Glycyrrhiza Glabra): A Phytochemical and Pharmacological Review," *Phytotherapy Research* 32, no. 12 (August 17, 2018): 2323–39, https://doi.org/10.1002/ptr.6178.

7. Michael Murray and Joseph Pizzorno, *The Encyclopedia of Natural Medicine* (New York: Atria Books, 2012).

8. Michael Murray and Joseph Pizzorno, *Textbook of Natural Medicine* (Philadelphia: Churchill Livingstone, 2020), 641–647.

9. A. R. Dehpour et al., "The Protective Effect of Liquorice Components and Their Derivatives Against Gastric Ulcer Induced By Aspirin in Rats," *Journal of Pharmacy and Pharmacology* 46, no. 2 (1994): 148–149, https://doi.org/10.1111/j.2042-7158.1994.tb03760.x.

10. C. Leite et al., "The Anti-Inflammatory Properties of Licorice (Glycyrrhiza Glabra)-Derived Compounds in Intestinal Disorders," *International Journal of Molecular Sciences* 23, no. 8 (2022): 4121, https://doi.org/10.3390/ijms23084121.

11. S. K. Murugan et al., "A Flavonoid Rich Standardized Extract of Glycyrrhiza Glabra Protects Intestinal Epithelial Barrier Function and Regulates the Tight-Junction Proteins Expression," *BMC Complementary Medicine and Therapies* 22, no. 1 (2022), https://doi.org/10.1186/s12906-021-03500-1.

12. W . W. Wang, S. Y. Qiao, and D. F. Li, "Amino Acids and Gut Function," *Amino Acids* 37, no. 1 (2009): 105–110, https://doi.org/10.1007/s00726-008-0152-4.

13. M. H. Kim and H. Kim, "The Roles of Glutamine in the Intestine and Its Implication in Intestinal Diseases," *International Journal of Molecular Sciences* 18, no. 5, (2017): 1051. https://doi.org/10.3390/ijms18051051.

14. S. Rastgoo et al, "Glutamine Supplementation Enhances the Effects of a Low Fodmap Diet in Irritable Bowel Syndrome Management," *Frontiers in Nutrition* 8 (2021), https://doi.org/10.3389/fnut.2021.746703.

15. N. Achamrah, P. Déchelotte, and M. Coëffier, "Glutamine and the Regulation of Intestinal Permeability," *Current Opinion in Clinical Nutrition & Metabolic Care* 20, no. 1 (2017): 86–91, https://doi.org/10.1097/mco.0000000000000339.

16. R. A. Potts et al. "Mast Cells and Histamine Alter Intestinal Permeability During Malaria Parasite Infection," *Immunobiology* 221, no. 3, (2016): 468–474, https://doi.org/10.1016/j.imbio.2015.11.003.

17. V. A. Uyanga et al., "Potential Implications of Citrulline and Quercetin on Gut Functioning of Monogastric Animals and Humans: A Comprehensive Review," *Nutrients* 13, no. 11 (2021): 3782, https://doi.org/10.3390/nu13113782.

18. Ibid.

19. T. Suzuki and H. Hara, "Quercetin Enhances Intestinal Barrier Function through the Assembly of Zonnula Occludens-2, Occludin, and Claudin-1 and the Expression of Claudin-4 in Caco-2 Cells," *The Journal of Nutrition* 139, no. 5 (2009): 965–974, https://doi.org/10.3945/jn.108.100867.

20. "Slippery elm," *Mount Sinai Health System*, accessed January 14, 2023, https://www.mountsinai.org/health-library/herb/slippery-elm.

21. Ibid.

22. L. Langmead et al., "Antioxidant effects of herbal therapies used by patients with inflammatory bowel disease: An *in vitro* study," *Alimentary Pharmacology & Therapeutics* 16 no. 2 (2002): 197–205, https://doi.org/10.1046/j.1365-2036.2002.01157.x.

23. Sharol Tilgner, "Marshmallow-Althea Officinalis," in *Herbal Medicine: From the Heart of the Earth* (Pleasant Hill, OR: Wise Acres, 2009), 86.

24. A. Deters et al. "Aqueous Extracts and Polysaccharides From Marshmallow Roots (Althea Officinalis L.): Cellular Internalisation and Stimulation of Cell Physiology of Human Epithelial Cells In Vitro," *Journal of Ethnopharmacology* 127, no. 1 (2010): 62–69, https://doi.org/10.1016/j.jep.2009.09.050.

25. S. S. Zaghlool et al., "Gastro-protective and Anti-oxidant Potential of Althaea officinalis and Solanum nigrum on Pyloric Ligation/indomethacin-induced Ulceration in Rats," *Antioxidants* 8, no. 11 (2019): 512, https://doi.org/10.3390/antiox8110512.

26. P. Riccio and R. Rossano, "Undigested Food and Gut Microbiota May Cooperate in the Pathogenesis of Neuroinflammatory Diseases: A Matter of Barriers and a Proposal on the Origin of Organ Specificity," *Nutrients* 11, no. 11 (2019): 2714, https://doi.org/10.3390/nu11112714

27. K. Saad et al., "A randomized, placebo-controlled trial of digestive enzymes in children with autism spectrum disorders," *Clinical Psychopharmacology and Neuroscience* 13, no. 2 (2015): 188–193, https://doi.org/10.9758/cpn.2015.13.2.188.

28. D. Y. Graham et al., "Enzyme Therapy for Functional Bowel Disease-Like Post-Prandial Distress," *Journal of Digestive Diseases* 19, no. 11 (2018): 650–656, https://doi.org/10.1111/1751-2980.12655.

29. S. Mills and K. Bone, "Principles of Herbal Pharmacology," in *Principles and Practice of Phytotherapy* (New York: Churchill Livingstone, 2000), 38–41.

30. M. K. McMullen, J. M. Whitehouse, and A. Towell, "Bitters: Time for a New Paradigm," *Evidence-Based Complementary and Alternative Medicine* 2015 (April 2015): 1–8, https://doi.org/10.1155/2015/670504.

31. P. Rezaie et al., "Effects of Bitter Substances on GI Function, Energy Intake and Glycaemia-Do Preclinical Findings Translate to Outcomes In Humans?" *Nutrients* 13, no. 4 (2021): 1317, https://doi.org/10.3390/nu13041317.

32. Ibid.

33. W. Buchwald, "Gentianae radix," in *The Gentianaceae, Volume 2: Biotechnology and Applications*, ed. P. Mikolajczak (Berlin: Springer-Verlag, 2015).

34. "Collagen: What It Is, Types, Function & Benefits," *Cleveland Clinic*, accessed January 15, 2023, https://my.clevelandclinic.org/health/articles /23089-collagen.

35. Harvard T.H. Chan School Of Public Health, "Collagen," *The Nutrition Source*, accessed January 15, 2023, https://www.hsph.harvard.edu/nutritionsource /collagen.

36. Cristiana Paul, Suzane Leser, and Steffen Oesser, "Significant Amounts of Functional Collagen Peptides Can Be Incorporated in the Diet While Maintaining Indispensable Amino Acid Balance," *Nutrients* 11, no. 5 (May 15, 2019): 1079, https://doi.org/10.3390/nu11051079.

37. W. Song et al., "Identification and Structure–Activity Relationship of Intestinal Epithelial Barrier Function Protective Collagen Peptides from Alaska Pollock Skin," *Marine Drugs* 17, no. 8 (2019): 450, https://doi.org /10.3390/md17080450

38. Katayoun Khoshbin and Michael Camilleri, "Effects of Dietary Components on Intestinal Permeability in Health and Disease," *American Journal Of Physiology: Gastrointestinal and Liver Physiology* 319, no. 5 (November 3, 2020), https://doi.org/10.1152/ajpgi.00245.2020.

39. "Vitamin A," *Linus Pauling Institute*, accessed January 3, 2023, https://lpi .oregonstate.edu/mic/vitamins/vitamin-A.

40. D. I. Thurnham et al., "Innate Immunity, Gut Integrity, and Vitamin A in Gambian and Indian Infants," *The Journal of Infectious Diseases* 182, no. s1 (September 2000), https://doi.org/10.1086/315912.

41. Lauge Kellermann et al., "Mucosal Vitamin D Signaling in Inflammatory Bowel Disease," *Autoimmunity Reviews* 19, no. 11 (2020): 102672, https://doi .org/10.1016/j.autrev.2020.102672.

42. Tara Raftery et al., "Effects of Vitamin D Supplementation on Intestinal Permeability, Cathelicidin and Disease Markers in Crohn's Disease: Results from a Randomised Double-Blind Placebo-Controlled Study," *United European Gastroenterology Journal* 3, no. 3 (June 2015): 294–302, https:// doi.org/10.1177/2050640615572176.

43. "Vitamin D," *NIH Office of Dietary Supplements*, last modified August 12, 2022, https://ods.od.nih.gov/factsheets/VitaminD-HealthProfessional.

44. "Zinc," *Linus Pauling Institute*, accessed January 3, 2023, https://lpi .oregonstate.edu/mic/minerals/zinc.

45. Sonja Skrovanek, "Zinc and Gastrointestinal Disease," *World Journal of Gastrointestinal Pathophysiology* 5, no. 4 (November 15, 2014): 496, https://doi.org/10.4291/wjgp.v5.i4.496.

46. Lara Costantini et al., "Impact of Omega-3 Fatty Acids on the Gut Microbiota," *International Journal of Molecular Sciences* 18, no. 12 (December 7, 2017): 2645, https://doi.org/10.3390/ijms18122645.

47. Francesca La Rosa et al., "The Gut-Brain Axis in Alzheimer's Disease and Omega-3. A Critical Overview of Clinical Trials," *Nutrients* 10, no. 9 (September 8, 2018): 1267, https://doi.org/10.3390/nu10091267.

Chapter 6

1. George Fink,. "Stress: The Health Epidemic of the 21st Century," Elsevier: SciTech Connect, April 26, 2016, https://scitechconnect.elsevier.com/stress-health-epidemic-21st-century.

2. Douglas S. Ramsay and Stephen C. Woods, "Clarifying the Roles of Homeostasis and Allostasis in Physiological Regulation," *Psychological Review* 121, no. 2 (April 2014): 225–47, https://doi.org/10.1037/a0035942.

3. Jenny Guidi et al., "Allostatic Load and Its Impact on Health: A Systematic Review," *Psychotherapy and Psychosomatics* 90, no. 1 (2020): 11–27, https://doi.org/10.1159/000510696.

4. Mark Stengler and Paul Anderson, "Contrasting Conventional and Integrative Oncology," Essay in *Outside the Box Cancer Therapies: Alternative Therapies That Treat and Prevent Cancer*, 1st ed., (Carlsbad, CA: Hay House, Inc., 2019), 41–43.

5. Habib Yaribeygi et al., "The Impact of Stress on Body Function: A Review," *ECLI Journal of Experimental and Clinical Sciences* 16 (July 2017): 1057–72, https://doi.org/10.17179/excli2017-480.

6. Committee on Herbal Medicinal Products, "Reflection Paper on the Adoptogenic Concept," *European Medicines Agency*, May 2008, https://www.ema.europa.eu/en/documents/scientific-guideline/reflection-paper-adaptogenic-concept_en.pdf.

7. K. Chandrasekhar, Jyoti Kapoor, and Sridhar Anishetty, "A Prospective, Randomized Double-Blind, Placebo-Controlled Study of Safety and Efficacy of a High-Concentration Full-Spectrum Extract of Ashwagandha Root in Reducing Stress and Anxiety in Adults," *Indian Journal of Psychological Medicine* 34, no. 3 (July 2012): 255–62, https://doi.org/10.4103/0253-7176.106022.

8. Ibid.

9. Yonghong Li et al., "Rhodiola Rosea L.: An Herb with Anti-Stress, Anti-Aging, and Immunostimulating Properties for Cancer Chemoprevention," *Current Pharmacology Reports* 3, no. 6 (September 14, 2017): 384–95, https://doi.org/10.1007/s40495-017-0106-1.

10. Ion-George Anghelescu et al., "Stress Management and the Role of *Rhodiola Rosea*: A Review," *International Journal of Psychiatry in Clinical Practice* 22, no. 4 (January 11, 2018): 242–52, https://doi.org/10.1080/13651501.2017.1417442.

11. Yi-Le Wu et al., "Association between Mthfr C677T Polymorphism and Depression: An Updated Meta-Analysis of 26 Studies," *Progress in Neuro-Psychopharmacology and Biological Psychiatry* 46 (July 4, 2013): 78–85, https://doi.org/10.1016/j.pnpbp.2013.06.015.

12. Hidetaka Hamasaki, "Effects of Diaphragmatic Breathing on Health: A Narrative Review," *Medicines* 7, no. 10 (October 15, 2020): 65, https://doi.org/10.3390/medicines7100065.

13. "Diaphragmatic Breathing Exercises," *Physiopedia*, accessed August 23, 2023. https://www.physio-pedia.com/Diaphragmatic_Breathing_Exercises.

14. Elizabeth F. Sutton et al., "Early Time-Restricted Feeding Improves Insulin Sensitivity, Blood Pressure, and Oxidative Stress Even without Weight Loss in Men with Prediabetes," *Cell Metabolism* 27, no. 6 (June 5, 2018), https://doi.org/10.1016/j.cmet.2018.04.010.

15. Anna Reade et al., "Toxic Chemicals," *Natural Resources Defense Council*, accessed February 7, 2022. https://www.nrdc.org/issues/toxic-chemicals.

16. James H. O'Keefe et al., "A Pesco-Mediterranean Diet with Intermittent Fasting," *Journal of the American College of Cardiology* 76, no. 12 (September 2020): 1484–93, https://doi.org/10.1016/j.jacc.2020.07.049.

17. Oliver Cameron Reddy and Ysbrand D. van der Werf, "The Sleeping Brain: Harnessing the Power of the Glymphatic System through Lifestyle Choices," *Brain Sciences* 10, no. 11 (November 17, 2020): 868, https://doi.org/10.3390/brainsci10110868.

18. Matthieu Clauss et al., "Interplay between Exercise and Gut Microbiome in the Context of Human Health and Performance," *Frontiers in Nutrition* 8 (June 10, 2021), https://doi.org/10.3389/fnut.2021.637010.

19. Zonghua Wang et al., "Gut Microbiota Associated with Effectiveness and Responsiveness to Mindfulness-Based Cognitive Therapy in Improving Trait Anxiety," *Frontiers in Cellular and Infection Microbiology* 12 (February 24, 2022), https://doi.org/10.3389/fcimb.2022.719829.

Chapter 7

1. Shingo Takashima et al., "Proton Pump Inhibitors Enhance Intestinal Permeability via Dysbiosis of Gut Microbiota under Stressed Conditions in Mice," *Neurogastroenterology & Motility* 32, no. 7 (April 21, 2020), https://doi.org/10.1111/nmo.13841.

2. Mark Stengler, "Risks of Proton Pump Inhibitors for Gastroesophageal Reflux Disease and a Diet Alternative," *Journal of Nutritional Health & Food Engineering* 10, no. 1 (April 28, 2020), https://doi.org/10.15406/jnhfe.2020.10.00338.

3. I. Mone et al., "Adherence to a Predominantly Mediterranean Diet Decreases the Risk of Gastroesophageal Reflux Disease: A Cross-Sectional Study in a South Eastern European Population," *Diseases of the Esophagus* 29, no. 7 (July 14, 2015): 794–800, https://doi.org/10.1111/dote.12384.

4. Giuseppe Antonio Malfa et al., "A Standardized Extract of Opuntia Ficus-Indica (L.) Mill and Olea Europaea L. Improves Gastrointestinal Discomfort: A Double-Blinded Randomized-Controlled Study," *Phytotherapy Research* 35, no. 7 (February 16, 2021): 3756–68, https://doi.org/10.1002/ptr.7074.

5. Jolanta Majka et al., "Melatonin in Prevention of the Sequence from Reflux Esophagitis to Barrett's Esophagus and Esophageal Adenocarcinoma: Experimental and Clinical Perspectives," *International Journal of Molecular Sciences* 19, no. 7 (July 13, 2018): 2033, https://doi.org/10.3390/ijms19072033.

6. Tharwat S. Kandil et al., "The Potential Therapeutic Effect of Melatonin in Gastro-Esophageal Reflux Disease," *BMC Gastroenterology* 10, no. 1 (January 18, 2010), https://doi.org/10.1186/1471-230x-10-7.

7. Jing Cheng and Arthur C. Ouwehand, "Gastroesophageal Reflux Disease and Probiotics: A Systematic Review," *Nutrients* 12, no. 1 (January 2, 2020): 132, https://doi.org/10.3390/nu12010132.

8. Carol A. Kumamoto, Mark S Gresnigt, and Bernhard Hube, "The Gut, the Bad and the Harmless: Candida Albicans as a Commensal and Opportunistic Pathogen in the Intestine," *Current Opinion in Microbiology* 56 (June 27, 2020): 7–15, https://doi.org/10.1016/j.mib.2020.05.006.

9. Laila Al-Ayadhi et al., "The Use of Biomarkers Associated with Leaky Gut as a Diagnostic Tool for Early Intervention in Autism Spectrum Disorder: A Systematic Review," *Gut Pathogens* 13, no. 1 (August 13, 2021), https://doi.org/10.1186/s13099-021-00448-y.

10. Louise Basmaciyan et al., "Candida Albicans Interactions with the Host: Crossing the Intestinal Epithelial Barrier," *Tissue Barriers* 7, no. 2 (June 12, 2019), https://doi.org/10.1080/21688370.2019.1612661.

11. Jun-Ke Wang et al., "Intestinal Mucosal Barrier in Functional Constipation: Dose It Change?" *World Journal of Clinical Cases* 10, no. 19 (July 6, 2022): 6385–98, https://doi.org/10.12998/wjcc.v10.i19.6385.

12. Toshifumi Ohkusa et al., "Gut Microbiota and Chronic Constipation: A Review and Update," *Frontiers in Medicine* 6 (February 12, 2019), https://doi.org/10.3389/fmed.2019.00019.

13. Lisa Vork et al., "Does Day-to-Day Variability in Stool Consistency Link to the Fecal Microbiota Composition?" *Frontiers in Cellular and Infection Microbiology* 11 (July 20, 2021), https://doi.org/10.3389/fcimb.2021.639667.

14. Eirini Dimidi et al., "Mechanisms of Action of Probiotics and the Gastrointestinal Microbiota on Gut Motility and Constipation," *Advances in Nutrition* 8, no. 3 (May 2017): 484–94, https://doi.org/10.3945/an.116.014407.

15. Wendy J. Dahl and Maria L. Stewart, "Position of the Academy of Nutrition and Dietetics: Health Implications of Dietary Fiber," *Journal of the Academy of Nutrition and Dietetics* 115, no. 11 (November 2015): 1861–70, https://doi .org/10.1016/j.jand.2015.09.003.

16. U.S. Department of Agriculture, "FoodData Central," last modified 2019, https://fdc.nal.usda.gov/index.html; USDA, "Food Sources of Dietary Fiber," *Dietary Guidelines for Americans*, accessed January 22, 2023, https://www. dietaryguidelines.gov/resources/2020-2025-dietary-guidelines-online-materials /food-sources-select-nutrients/food-0; Wendy J. Dahl and Maria L. Stewart, "Position of the Academy of Nutrition and Dietetics: Health Implications of Dietary Fiber," *Journal of the Academy of Nutrition and Dietetics* 115, no. 11 (November 2015): 1861–70, https://doi.org/10.1016/j.jand.2015.09.003.

17. Aleksandra Tarasiuk et al., "Triphala: Current Applications and New Perspectives on the Treatment of Functional Gastrointestinal Disorders," *Chinese Medicine* 13, no. 1 (July 18, 2018), https://doi.org/10.1186 /s13020-018-0197-6.

18. "Definition & Facts for Gallstones," *National Institute of Diabetes and Digestive and Kidney Diseases*, last modified November 2017, https://www.niddk.nih .gov/health-information/digestive-diseases/gallstones/definition-facts.

19. Irina N. Grigor'eva and Tatyana I. Romanova, "Gallstone Disease and Microbiome," *Microorganisms* 8, no. 6 (June 2, 2020): 835, https://doi .org/10.3390/microorganisms8060835.

20. K. J. Dabos et al., "The Effect of Mastic Gum on Helicobacter Pylori: A Randomized Pilot Study," *Phytomedicine* 17, no. 3–4 (March 2010): 296–99, https://doi.org/10.1016/j.phymed.2009.09.010.

21. K. J. Dabos et al., "Is Chios Mastic Gum Effective in the Treatment of Functional Dyspepsia? A Prospective Randomised Double-Blind Placebo Controlled Trial," *Journal of Ethnopharmacology* 127, no. 2 (February 3, 2010): 205–9, https://doi.org/10.1016/j.jep.2009.11.021.

22. A. G. Morgan et al., "Comparison between Cimetidine and Caved-s in the Treatment of Gastric Ulceration, and Subsequent Maintenance Therapy," *Gut* 23, no. 6 (June 1, 1982): 545–51, https://doi.org/10.1136/gut.23.6.545.

23. Susan Hewlings and Douglas Kalman, "A Review of Zinc-L-Carnosine and Its Positive Effects on Oral Mucositis, Taste Disorders, and Gastrointestinal Disorders," *Nutrients* 12, no. 3 (February 29, 2020): 665, https://doi.org /10.3390/nu12030665.

24. Masoud Keikha and Mohsen Karbalaei, "Probiotics as the Live Microscopic Fighters against Helicobacter Pylori Gastric Infections," *BMC Gastroenterology* 21, no. 1 (October 20, 2021), https://doi.org/10.1186/s12876-021-01977-1.

25. Ibid.

26. "The Specific Carbohydrate Diet - Stanford Medicine," *North American Society for Pediatric Gastroenterology, Hepatology and Nutrition (NASPGHAN)*, accessed July 29, 2023, https://med.stanford.edu/content/dam/sm/gastroenterology /documents/IBD/CarbDiet%20PDF%20final.pdf.

27. Arjun Gandhi et al., "Methane Positive Small Intestinal Bacterial Overgrowth in Inflammatory Bowel Disease and Irritable Bowel Syndrome: A Systematic Review and Meta-Analysis," *Gut Microbes* 13, no. 1 (June 30, 2021), https://doi.org/10.1080/19490976.2021.1933313.

28. Sophia J. Oak and Rajesh Jha, "The Effects of Probiotics in Lactose Intolerance: A Systematic Review," *Critical Reviews in Food Science and Nutrition* 59, no. 11 (February 9, 2018): 1675–83, https://doi.org/10.1080/10408398.2018.1425977.

Chapter 8

1. I. Salem et al., "The Gut Microbiome as a Major Regulator of the Gut-Skin Axis," *Frontiers in Microbiology* 9 (2018): 1459, https://doi.org/10.3389/fmicb.2018.01459.

2. "Skin Conditions by the Numbers," *American Academy of Dermatology*, accessed August 23, 2023. https://www.aad.org/media/stats-numbers.

3. Y. B. Lee et al., "Potential Role of the Microbiome in Acne: A Comprehensive Review," *Journal of Clinical Medicine* 8, no.7 (2019): 987, https://doi.org/10.3390/jcm8070987.

4. Jessica Cervantes et al., "The Role of Zinc in the Treatment of Acne: A Review of the Literature," *Dermatologic Therapy* 31, no. 1 (November 28, 2017), https://doi.org/10.1111/dth.12576.

5. Harsimran Kaur Malhi et al., "Tea Tree Oil Gel for Mild to Moderate Acne; a 12 Week Uncontrolled, Open-Label Phase II Pilot Study," *Australasian Journal of Dermatology* 58, no. 3 (August 2017): 205–10, https://doi.org/10.1111/ajd.12465.

6. Azadeh Goodarzi et al., "The Potential of Probiotics for Treating Acne Vulgaris: A Review of Literature on Acne and Microbiota," *Dermatologic Therapy* 33, no. 3 (April 7, 2020), https://doi.org/10.1111/dth.13279.

7. K. Chandrasekhar, Jyoti Kapoor, and Sridhar Anishetty, "A Prospective, Randomized Double-Blind, Placebo-Controlled Study of Safety and Efficacy of a High-Concentration Full-Spectrum Extract of Ashwagandha Root in Reducing Stress and Anxiety in Adults," *Indian Journal of Psychological Medicine* 34, no. 3 (July 2012): 255–62, https://doi.org/10.4103/0253-7176.106022.

8. Ion-George Anghelescu et al., "Stress Management and the Role of Rhodiola Rosea: A Review," *International Journal of Psychiatry in Clinical Practice* 22, no. 4 (January 11, 2018): 242–52, https://doi.org/10.1080/13651501.2017.1417442.

9. "Allergy Facts," *Asthma & Allergy Foundation of America*, accessed November 14, 2022. https://aafa.org/allergies/allergy-facts.

10. A. M. Watts et al., "The Gut Microbiome of Adults with Allergic Rhinitis Is Characterised by Reduced Diversity and an Altered Abundance of Key

Microbial Taxa Compared to Controls," *International Archives of Allergy and Immunology* 182, no. 2 (2021): 94–105: https://doi.org/10.1159/000510536.

11. Cezmi A. Akdis, "Does the Epithelial Barrier Hypothesis Explain the Increase in Allergy, Autoimmunity and Other Chronic Conditions?" *Nature Reviews Immunology* 21, no. 11 (November 2021): 739–51, https://doi.org/10.1038/s41577-021-00538-7.

12. "Asthma," *Asthma & Allergy Foundation of America*, accessed January 17, 2023, https://aafa.org/asthma.

13. Alessio Fasano, "Zonulin and Its Regulation of Intestinal Barrier Function: The Biological Door to Inflammation, Autoimmunity, and Cancer," *Physiological Reviews* 91, no. 1 (2011): 151–75, https://doi.org/10.1152/physrev.00003.2008.

14. S. Yamada et al., "Effects of Repeated Oral Intake of a Quercetin-Containing Supplement on Allergic Reaction: a Randomized, Placebo-Controlled, Double-Blind Parallel-Group Study," *European Review for Medical and Pharmacological Sciences* 26, no. 12 (June 2022): 4331–45, https://doi.org/10.26355/eurrev_202206_29072.

15. Maria R. Cesarone et al., "Supplementary Prevention and Management of Asthma with Quercetin Phytosome: A Pilot Registry," *Minerva Medica* 110, no. 6 (December 2019), https://doi.org/10.23736/s0026-4806.19.06319-5.

16. Benjamin H. S. Lau et al., "Pycnogenol® as an Adjunct in the Management of Childhood Asthma," *Journal of Asthma* 41, no. 8 (July 2009): 825–32, https://doi.org/10.1081/jas-200038433.

17. M. Clapp et al., "Gut Microbiota's Effect on Mental Health: The Gut-Brain Axis," *Clinics and Practice* 7, no. 4 (2017): 987, https://doi.org/10.4081/cp.2017.987.

18. Piril Hepsomali et al., "Effects of Oral Gamma-Aminobutyric Acid (GABA) Administration on Stress and Sleep in Humans: A Systematic Review," *Frontiers in Neuroscience* 14 (September 17, 2020), https://doi.org/10.3389/fnins.2020.00923.

19. Jackson L. Williams et al., "The Effects of Green Tea Amino Acid L-Theanine Consumption on the Ability to Manage Stress and Anxiety Levels: A Systematic Review," *Plant Foods for Human Nutrition* 75, no. 1 (November 22, 2019): 12–23, https://doi.org/10.1007/s11130-019-00771-5.

20. Mark Stengler, "A Review of the Mechanisms and Clinical Effects of CBD for Neurological Conditions," *Journal of Neurology and Stroke* 11, no. 4 (August 2, 2021): 110-1, https://medcraveonline.com/JNSK/JNSK-11-00466.pdf.

21. Anna-Maria Orbai, "What Are Common Symptoms of Autoimmune Disease?" *Johns Hopkins Medicine*, last modified July 22, 2022, https://www.hopkinsmedicine.org/health/wellness-and-prevention/what-are-common-symptoms-of-autoimmune-disease.

22. Cezmi A. Akdis, "Does the Epithelial Barrier Hypothesis Explain the Increase in Allergy, Autoimmunity and Other Chronic Conditions?" *Nature Reviews Immunology* 21, no. 11 (November 12, 2021): 739–51, https://doi.org/10.1038/s41577-021-00538-7.

23. Albert Shieh et al., "Gut Permeability, Inflammation, and Bone Density across the Menopause Transition," *JCI Insight* 5, no. 2 (December 12, 2019), https://doi.org/10.1172/jci.insight.134092.

24. A. G. Nilsson et al., "Lactobacillus Reuteri Reduces Bone Loss in Older Women with Low Bone Mineral Density: A Randomized, Placebo-Controlled, Double-Blind, Clinical Trial," *Journal of Internal Medicine* 284, no. 3 (June 21, 2018): 307–17, https://doi.org/10.1111/joim.12805.

25. Rachel H. X. Wong et al., "Regular Supplementation with Resveratrol Improves Bone Mineral Density in Postmenopausal Women: A Randomized, Placebo-controlled Trial," *Journal of Bone and Mineral Research* 35, no. 11 (June 14, 2020): 2121–31, https://doi.org/10.1002/jbmr.4115.

26. M. Clapp et al., "Gut Microbiota's Effect on Mental Health: The Gut-Brain Axis," *Clinics and Practice* 7, no. 4 (2017): 987, https://doi.org/10.4081/cp.2017.987.

27. Wolfgang Marx et al., "Effect of Saffron Supplementation on Symptoms of Depression and Anxiety: A Systematic Review and Meta-Analysis," *Nutrition Reviews* 77, no. 8 (May 28, 2019): 557–71, https://doi.org/10.1093/nutrit/nuz023.

28. Wenting Xie et al., "Glucose-Lowering Effect of Berberine on Type 2 Diabetes: A Systematic Review and Meta-Analysis," *Frontiers in Pharmacology* 13 (November 16, 2022), https://doi.org/10.3389/fphar.2022.1015045.

29. Roger Steigerwalt et al., "Pycnogenol Improves Microcirculation, Retinal Edema, and Visual Acuity in Early Diabetic Retinopathy," *Journal of Ocular Pharmacology and Therapeutics* 25, no. 6 (December 2009): 537–40, https://doi.org/10.1089/jop.2009.0023.

30. "Eczema Types: Atopic Dermatitis Causes," *American Academy of Dermatology*, last modified November 11, 2022, https://www.aad.org/public/diseases/eczema/types/atopic-dermatitis/causes.

31. M. Niewiem and U. Grzybowska-Chlebowczyk, "Intestinal Barrier Permeability in Allergic Diseases," *Nutrients* 14, no. 9 (2022): 1893. https://doi.org/10.3390/nu14091893.

32. Ibid.

33. E. Rusu et al., "Prebiotics and Probiotics in Atopic Dermatitis," *Experimental and Therapeutic Medicine* 18, no. 2 (2019): 926–931. https://doi.org/10.3892/etm.2019.7678.

34. Leonardo César Cayres et al., "Detection of Alterations in the Gut Microbiota and Intestinal Permeability in Patients with Hashimoto Thyroiditis," *Frontiers in Immunology* 12 (March 5, 2021), https://doi.org/10.3389/fimmu.2021.579140.

35. S. Benvenga et al., "The Role of Inositol in Thyroid Physiology and in Subclinical Hypothyroidism Management," *Frontiers in Endocrinology* 12 (2021): 1–13, https://doi.org/10.3389/fendo.2021.662582.

36. The American Academy of Sleep Medicine, "Insomnia," accessed July 29, 2023, https://aasm.org/resources/factsheets/insomnia.pdf.

37. Y. Li et al., "The Role of Microbiome in Insomnia, Circadian Disturbance and Depression," *Frontiers in Psychiatry* 9 (2018), https://doi.org/10.3389/fpsyt.2018.00669.

38. R. P. Smith et al., "Gut Microbiome Diversity Is Associated with Sleep Physiology in Humans," *PloS One* 14, no. 10 (2019): e0222394, https://doi.org/10.1371/journal.pone.0222394.

39. Osteoarthritis Action Alliance, "OA Prevalence and Burden," OA Modules, last modified October 12, 2022, https://oaaction.unc.edu/oa-module/oa-prevalence-and-burden.

40. Nicola Veronese et al., "Glucosamine Sulphate: An Umbrella Review of Health Outcomes," *Therapeutic Advances in Musculoskeletal Disease* 12 (2020), https://doi.org/10.1177/1759720x20975927.

41. James P. Lugo, Zainulabedin M. Saiyed, and Nancy E. Lane, "Efficacy and Tolerability of an Undenatured Type II Collagen Supplement in Modulating Knee Osteoarthritis Symptoms: A Multicenter Randomized, Double-Blind, Placebo-Controlled Study," *Nutrition Journal* 15, no. 1 (January 29, 2015), https://doi.org/10.1186/s12937-016-0130-8.

42. Bénédicte M.J. Merle et al., "Mediterranean Diet and Incidence of Advanced Age-Related Macular Degeneration," *Ophthalmology* 126, no. 3 (March 2019): 381–90, https://doi.org/10.1016/j.ophtha.2018.08.006.

43. Tatjana Rundek et al., "Gut Permeability and Cognitive Decline: A Pilot Investigation in the Northern Manhattan Study," *Brain, Behavior, & Immunity - Health* 12 (March 2021): 100214, https://doi.org/10.1016/j.bbih.2021.100214.

44. Ibid.

45. Eri Nakazaki et al., "Citicoline and Memory Function in Healthy Older Adults: A Randomized, Double-Blind, Placebo-Controlled Clinical Trial," *The Journal of Nutrition* 151, no. 8 (August 7, 2021): 2153–60, https://doi.org/10.1093/jn/nxab119.

46. Chuenjid Kongkeaw et al., "Meta-Analysis of Randomized Controlled Trials on Cognitive Effects of Bacopa Monnieri Extract." *Journal of Ethnopharmacology* 151, no. 1 (2014): 528–35, https://doi.org/10.1016/j.jep.2013.11.008.

47. Albert Shieh et al., "Gut Permeability, Inflammation, and Bone Density across the Menopause Transition," *JCI Insight* 5, no. 2 (December 12, 2019), https://doi.org/10.1172/jci.insight.134092.

48. Sradhanjali Mohapatra et al., "Benefits of Black Cohosh (CIMICIFUGA Racemosa) for Women Health: An up-Close and in-Depth Review," *Pharmaceuticals* 15, no. 3 (February 23, 2022): 278, https://doi.org/10.3390/ph15030278.

49. H. O. Meissner, A. Mscisz, and H. Reich-Bilinska, "Hormone-Balancing Effect of Pre-Gelatinized Organic Maca (Lepidium Peruvianum Chacon): (II) Physiological and Symptomatic Responses of Early-Postmenopausal Women to Standardized Doses of Maca in Double Blind, Randomized,

Placebo-Controlled, Multi-Centre Clinical Study," *International Journal of Biomedical Science* 2, no. 4 (n.d.).

50. Ilona Hasper et al., "Long-Term Efficacy and Safety of the Special Extract ERR 731 of Rheum Rhaponticum in Perimenopausal Women with Menopausal Symptoms," *Menopause* 16, no. 1 (2009): 117–31, https://doi.org/10.1097/gme.0b013e3181806446.

51. Stephanie S. Faubion et al., "The 2022 Hormone Therapy Position Statement of the North American Menopause Society," *Menopause* 29, no. 7 (2022): 767–794, https://doi.org/10.1097/gme.0000000000002028.

52. T. Takeda et al., "Characteristics of the Gut Microbiota in Women with Premenstrual Symptoms: A Cross-Sectional Study," *PloS One* 17, no. 5 (2022): e0268466, https://doi.org/10.1371/journal.pone.0268466.

53. Raphael O. Cerqeuira, Benica N. Frey, and Elisa Brietzke, "Vitex Agnus Castus for Premenstrual Syndrome and Premenstrual Dysphoric Disorder: A Systematic Review," *Archives of Women's Mental Health* 20, no. 6 (December 2017), https://doi.org/10.1007/s00737-017-0791-0.

54. Miriam C. De Souza et al., "A Synergistic Effect of a Daily Supplement for 1 Month of 200 Mg Magnesium plus 50 Mg Vitamin B6 for the Relief of Anxiety-Related Premenstrual Symptoms: A Randomized, Double-Blind, Crossover Study," *Journal of Women's Health & Gender-Based Medicine* 9, no. 2 (March 2000): 131–39, https://doi.org/10.1089/152460900318623.

55. Ibid.

56. Mina Taghiabadi et al., "Beneficial Role of Calcium in Premenstrual Syndrome: A Systematic Review of Current Literature," *International Journal of Preventive Medicine* 11, no. 1 (September 22, 2020), https://doi.org/10.4103/ijpvm.ijpvm_243_19.

57. "Psoriasis: Causes," American Academy of Dermatology, accessed August 23, 2023, https://www.aad.org/public/diseases/psoriasis/what/causes.

58. K. Polak et al., "Psoriasis and Gut Microbiome—Current State of Art," *International journal of Molecular Sciences* 22, no. 9 (2021): 4529, https://doi.org/10.3390/ijms22094529.

59. P. Haines Ely, "Is Psoriasis a Bowel Disease? Successful Treatment with Bile Acids and Bioflavonoids Suggests It Is," *Clinics in Dermatology* 36, no. 3 (2018): 376–89, https://doi.org/10.1016/j.clindermatol.2018.03.011.

60. Ranju Pokharel et al. "Assessment of Vitamin D Level in Patients with Psoriasis and Its Correlation with Disease Severity: A Case–Control Study," *Psoriasis: Targets and Therapy* Volume 12 (September 13, 2022): 251–58, https://doi.org/10.2147/ptt.s369426.

61. H. Joung and D. M., "Serum Level of Sex Steroid Hormone Is Associated with Diversity And Profiles of Human Gut Microbiome," *Research in Microbiology* 170, no. 4–5 (2019): 192–201, https://doi.org/10.1016/j.resmic.2019.03.003

62. Sanjaya Chauhan, Manoj K. Srivastava, and Anklesh K. Pathak, "Effect of Standardized Root Extract of Ashwagandha (*Withania Somnifera*) on Well-being and Sexual Performance in Adult Males: A Randomized Controlled

Trial," *Health Science Reports* 5, no. 4 (July 20, 2022), https://doi.org/10.1002/hsr2.741.

63. Talbott et al., "Effect of Tongkat Ali"; Ralf R. Henkel et al., "Tongkat Ali as a Potential Herbal Supplement for Physically Active Male and Female Seniors—a Pilot Study," *Phytotherapy Research* 28, no. 4 (2013): 544–50, https://doi.org/10.1002/ptr.5017.

64. Gianluca Scuderi, Emidio Troiani, and Angelo Maria Minnella, "Gut Microbiome in Retina Health: The Crucial Role of the Gut-Retina Axis," *Frontiers in Microbiology* 12 (January 14, 2022), https://doi.org/10.3389/fmicb.2021.726792.

65. Yuji Morita, Kenta Jounai, Mika Miyake, Masaharu Inaba, and Osamu Kanauchi, "Effect of Heat-Killed Lactobacillus Paracasei KW3110 Ingestion on Ocular Disorders Caused by Visual Display Terminal (VDT) Loads: A Randomized, Double-Blind, Placebo-Controlled Parallel-Group Study," *Nutrients* 10, no. 8 (August 9, 2018): 1058, https://doi.org/10.3390/nu10081058.

INDEX

ACKNOWLEDGMENTS

My thanks to Reid Tracy, Lara Asher, Nicolette Salamanca Young, and the team at Hay House for their support of this cutting-edge book. Also, thanks to Dr. Jared Zeff, who emphasized in my holistic medical training more than 30 years ago the fundamental importance of treating digestive health as a root cause of most illnesses. In addition, thank you to my friend and colleague Dr. Steve Nenninger, an expert in treating digestive ailments, who has supported my work since our days in medical school. And I cannot thank enough my very patient wife, Dr. Angela Stengler, for her support with my seemingly endless projects of passion. And most importantly, gratitude to the One we read about in John 1:3, who is the master engineer behind the incredibly complex digestive system and body.

ABOUT THE AUTHOR

Dr. Mark Stengler is a naturopathic medical doctor in private practice in Encinitas, California. He is a best-selling author and has authored over 20 books, including *Prescription for Natural Cures*, *Outside the Box Cancer Therapies*, and *Healing the Prostate*. He has integrative and functional medicine expertise, combining the best of conventional and natural medicine. He was chosen as Doctor of the Year in 2019 and Doctor of the Decade in 2021 by the International Association of Top Professionals. In 2022, he was selected as Top California Doctor by *Top Doctor Magazine*. In 2023, Dr. Stengler was chosen as Top Naturopathic Medical Doctor by FindaTopDoc. You can visit Dr. Stengler online at **www.markstengler.com**.

Hay House Titles of Related Interest

YOU CAN HEAL YOUR LIFE, the movie,
starring Louise Hay & Friends
(available as an online streaming video)
www.hayhouse.com/louise-movie

THE SHIFT, the movie,
starring Dr. Wayne W. Dyer
(available as an online streaming video)
www.hayhouse.com/the-shift-movie

∘ ∘ ⊚ ∘ ∘

*Beyond Longevity: A Proven Plan for Healing Faster, Feeling Better,
and Thriving at Any Age*, by Jason Prall

*Eat for Energy: How to Beat Fatigue, Supercharge Your Mitochondria,
and Unlock All-Day Energy*, by Ari Whitten

Real Superfoods: Everyday Ingredients to Elevate Your Health,
by Ocean Robbins and Nichole Dandrea-Russert

*Whole Brain Living: The Anatomy of Choice and the Four Characters
That Drive Our Life*, by Jill Bolte Taylor

All of the above are available at your local bookstore,
or may be ordered by contacting Hay House (see next page).

∘ ∘ ⊚ ∘ ∘

We hope you enjoyed this Hay House book. If you'd like to receive our online catalog featuring additional information on Hay House books and products, or if you'd like to find out more about the Hay Foundation, please contact:

Hay House, Inc., P.O. Box 5100, Carlsbad, CA 92018-5100
(760) 431-7695 or (800) 654-5126
(760) 431-6948 (fax) or (800) 650-5115 (fax)
www.hayhouse.com® • www.hayfoundation.org

———

Published in Australia by: Hay House Australia Pty. Ltd.,
18/36 Ralph St., Alexandria NSW 2015
Phone: 612-9669-4299 • *Fax:* 612-9669-4144
www.hayhouse.com.au

Published in the United Kingdom by: Hay House UK, Ltd.,
The Sixth Floor, Watson House, 54 Baker Street, London W1U 7BU
Phone: +44 (0)20 3927 7290 • *Fax:* +44 (0)20 3927 7291
www.hayhouse.co.uk

Published in India by: Hay House Publishers India,
Muskaan Complex, Plot No. 3, B-2, Vasant Kunj, New Delhi 110 070
Phone: 91-11-4176-1620 • *Fax:* 91-11-4176-1630
www.hayhouse.co.in

———

Access New Knowledge.
Anytime. Anywhere.

Learn and evolve at your own pace
with the world's leading experts.

www.hayhouseU.com

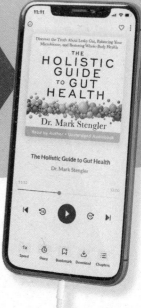